ALL ABOUT CLINICAL RESEARCH:

WORD SEARCH AND FLASH CARDS FOR ICH GUIDELINES FOR GOOD CLINICAL PRACTICE

(TRAVEL SIZE 2ND EDITION)

A STUDY GUIDE FOR THE
INTERNATIONAL COUNCIL FOR HARMONISATION OF TECHNICAL
REQUIREMENTS FOR REGISTRATION OF PHARMACEUTICALS FOR
HUMAN USE (ICH) GUIDELINES FOR GOOD CLINICAL PRACTICE
[E6 (R2) – THE INTEGRATED ADDENDUM TO E6(R1)]

SOLAR BIOMEDICAL

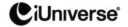

ALL ABOUT CLINICAL RESEARCH: WORD SEARCH AND FLASH CARDS FOR ICH GUIDELINES FOR GOOD CLINICAL PRACTICE (TRAVEL SIZE 2ND EDITION) A STUDY GUIDE FOR THE INTERNATIONAL COUNCIL FOR HARMONISATION OF TECHNICAL REQUIREMENTS FOR REGISTRATION OF PHARMACEUTICALS FOR HUMAN USE (ICH) GUIDELINES FOR GOOD CLINICAL PRACTICE [E6 (R2) – THE INTEGRATED ADDENDUM TO E6(R1)]

iUniverse books may be ordered through booksellers or by contacting:

iUniverse
1663 Liberty Drive
Bloomington, IN 47403
www.iuniverse.com
844-349-9409

Because of the dynamic nature of the Internet, any web addresses or links contained in this book may have changed since publication and may no longer be valid. The views expressed in this work are solely those of the author and do not necessarily reflect the views of the publisher, and the publisher hereby disclaims any responsibility for them.

Any people depicted in stock imagery provided by Getty Images are models, and such images are being used for illustrative purposes only. Certain stock imagery © Getty Images.

ISBN: 978-1-6632-4991-3 (sc)
ISBN: 978-1-6632-4992-0 (e)

Library of Congress Control Number: 2023900865

Print information available on the last page.

iUniverse rev. date: 02/07/2023

CONTENTS

FOREWORD

Some of the most successful educational practices utilized throughout the United States and United Kingdom are based on accelerated learning techniques (brain games), such as word search and crossword puzzles. When used effectively, these techniques have been reported by learners to make them feel more independent and achieve good results. Teachers have reported evidence of improved institutional ethos and increased learner participation.

Word searches and puzzles are fun, easy, and great exercises for the brain. They require the learner to focus, think, and work toward getting results. It is our hope that this book will serve as a fun and successful study tool for all persons entering the industry as new clinical research professionals, as well as for experienced clinical research professionals preparing to take their certification exams.

Solar Biomedical is dedicated to creating practical and innovative ways of bringing clinical research training to novice and experienced clinical research professionals. The company's experience in training and monitoring phases I–IV clinical trials affords it over sixteen years of successful outcomes in those areas. The company is backed by clinical research professionals with scientific and advanced degrees in the biological and applied sciences as well as in the educational arts.

HOW TO USE THIS BOOK

It is important to understand that the standards for conducting clinical trials can be divided into two categories: (1) The laws and (2) The rules. Certification exams and daily clinical research practices are based on these two standards. *The laws* for conducting clinical research trials are enforceable government regulations and are country specific. The laws can be found in a country's local registries. However, *the rules* for conducting clinical research trials are guidelines created to facilitate the integrity and acceptance of a clinical trial's data globally. These rules are found in the International Council for Harmonisation of Technical Requirements for Pharmaceuticals for Human Use (ICH) Guidelines for Good Clinical Practice (GCP), and serve as a uniform global guide for all research professionals to follow. The purpose of this book is to provide clinical research professionals with a fun and effective way of learning and remembering the information found in ICH Guidelines for Good Clinical Practice through word searches and flash cards.

- Use the ***word search activities*** to help with word associations to help focus and learn the different parts of the ICH Guidelines for Good Clinical Practice. Guidelines [E6 (R2)] as published at Step 4 of the ICH process in version dated November 9, 2016, [E8 (R1)] as published at Step 4 of the ICH process in version dated October 6, 2021, and Clinical Safety Data Management (E2A) as published in the U.S. Federal Register March 1, 1995 are attached to this book for your easy reference when solving the word search puzzles.
- Use the ***flash cards*** as a tool for remembering specific GCP rules in clinical research.

WORD SEARCHES

Safety Is the Name of the Game

*(Find each **bolded** word in the word search below.)*

Good **clinical practice** (GCP) is an **international ethical** and **scientific quality standard** for **designing**, **conducting**, **recording**, and **reporting trials** that **involve** the **participation** of human subjects. Compliance with this standard provides public assurance that the **rights**, **safety**, and well-being of trial subjects are **protected**; consistent with the **principles** that have their **origin** in the Declaration of Helsinki, and that the clinical trial data are **credible**.

G I S I N C E T I L S C E H D I G P T T S T A R T
D I E O I I L Y I I C V S A I E R S R P N C T R E E T G I
N L L R Y O B E R E A S L N L V T S C A I E E O T H
O G T L P R T G I R G Q L S A I N R C I D P C A P S T
G I C I L I R D E O T C I A T V I C A G L V C R E E
I E C I L I E N R I S I R C T Y A D P N T L I I N G
E D E N I A D R E T S S C O R N O S I V G I I D O I A
D G I I U E C P O S N A Z D O N E R Z P C N C R C I E
P R O Q O O L Z Q C L O R Z N T S T E I U Y G L E
E L P S R Z I A G R I T S D G U A Z H C D P L I O
D A T D C Z I V L R I O O S N I C R S I T R C Z V
E I S I O P O R T S D I I T P I T A C C E T A F
T Z A Z H I S T R R O L Z C I C F L T D C C R A P I E
G T R A A T R S T A Z D A R D T I Y R C C Z R L P E
Z Z O C L A R A I T Z T Q I I F T L D O A T I I Z
R V C O L P G Z I T R O P P E R A Z A E C O O Z E C
A S Z Z I I T T Z Z R T D C C T E C T A C O S R E S
E H I D I C T T H O I O C C V C I I C V I R R E C
I H J L I R I G G A P O I C C Z E Z I A C V E S
Z G D C E T A R Z S Z E I L C E S I T O C G I L Z
O I Z T E R Z A T I O Z A L C T I L O P R Z I O I
R R L I G A S Z F Q I E A P R L A C R I U I E V A
A I L Z Z P I S Y T E F A S C E I E P P C Z G Z G
S R G E E O T C I R R P R L L H C O C G I P Z S I Z
Q Z D A Z I R Z E R I I D A R B E V R C O E E L Z

Can I Ever Throw Away Essential Documents?

GCP 4.9.5and 5.5.12

*(Find each **bolded** word in the word search below.)*

Essential documents should be **retained** until at least two years after the last approval of a **marketing application** in an **ICH-region** and until there are no pending or **contemplated** marketing applications in an ICH region or at least two **years** have **elapsed** since the formal discontinuation of clinical development of the investigational product. These documents should be retained for a longer period, however, if required by the applicable regulatory **requirements** or by an **agreement** with the sponsor. It is the **responsibility** of the sponsor to inform the investigator/institution as to when these documents no longer need to be retained.

```
A D G L I U A A M U E O E C R L S E R E N S E E M
I S I C E C C M S I T E E L C T O I L A U G E E I
K A G E D I M N E M E S D S B C P A S D I A M G K
E R M C C L N E A R E N I S E N N P S Y G N I M O
E Y M E R E Q N R N E N P S Y O G O L E Y D G K E L
T P L S T R E S P O N S I B I L I T Y E D S I I
R L A C M S S T M O U C M S N G I C S C I E E E M
P P S G E N C A L R E Q U I R E M E N T S S T L I
Y I I B Y R N R L O S I D R R M L L Y P T T P
E L R E P R O S G C G I I E H S O N T A A I T G
S N A A E Q N I I T E N S P E C R I E I L L T O P
E E R A I E N T R N N M L T E I I E M T I E A E E
E S R M E P I A L L G E A C O M N S M N R A I D N
M S S S P E T C S M E S M R L C U E R I Q S O I S
D I S E E C D I U E E T E U K M C E N I T R P D E E I
I T T D N L S L P E E B M T I C E I D D R D R E Y N
N K A R K T E P T R M S K M T O T A I H T C B S Y
A S D H N U I P R G I E L P D E D I E B S Q R I D
N E I R I Q E A U A T E L M T L I N N O R E E E R
Y I S E Y T S R L L I E M E U A R R C G M E N T S
M M G D S T R A A T C Q A L P E I E M T P A T R N N
N C G O N T E M P L A T E D T P O I N K S U E O P L
D Q P G R G T D E N I A T E R Y P S Y S E R N T N
U P L K N C A E I T I U T R E E E T E A S R E E
O I N E N E P N I I P D S M I N I E D U E N A S E
```

Names of Documents Found in Both the 21 CFRs for Clinical Research and the ICH/GCP Guidelines

(Find each word in the word search below.)

AMENDMENTS
ANNUALREPORT
CASEREPORTFORM
CURRICULUMVITAE
EXPEDITEDREPORT
IRBAPPROVALS
PROGRESSREPORT
PROTOCOLS
SAFETYREPORT
SHIPPINGRECORDS
SOURCEDOCUMENTS

Knowing the Signs and Symptoms

GCP 1.2

*(Find each **bolded** word in the word search below.)*

An **adverse event** can be any **unfavorable** and **unintended sign** (including an **abnormal laboratory** finding), **symptom**, or **disease** temporarily **associated** with the use of a **medicinal** (**investigational**) **product**, whether or not related to the medicinal (investigational) product. (See also the ICH **Guideline** for **Clinical Safety Data Management**: Definitions and Standards for Expedited Reporting.)

```
S V A M L A N Y D N L A L L I I Y R Z N O C A E E
U N L N A I T N D A M I A G U Y V V M L R S U I D A
N S M E S R D T A A O R B I C T P I V U A T T T T
N A A O T C S A U T T O E S I C N I E D G I S Z N
A D U B I T O M V T P T R T U T E E A L D E I Z M
S A S E I A O S N G M L A B L L N O I U R C D T T
I I R N E S E A L G Y N T U B I G N E I A N S E C
G A A S O N I I O N S M O N T A U T M A D A S T I C
N A U A A E I N L A N I R S E R I E T E T R E A S
B G N M I R R V I E O E Y S T V D E E N E O N N Y
C C G N M N P E G I R M L A D I E O T V A N L V T
N N I R I R O S U A A M N S C I L M D E I G D L G
O C S I O S I T E N O G T I G T I A D D L N I M M
E U L D U D L I A U D D N P N A N F E A A S N A I
N C U I L A O G M G U A A Y E T E D C D M S S D T
A C S G D N E A L A L A G T G S N I I N R S I C O T
T V A C N M N T N O T N I S A E N U G F O I N T T
M R F V E N G I C F D V A A T I A S I C N M E N A
A E N G E T O L A R A O N L R E P I I B S T Z A
M M T A C N N N I T I C I D S A E S A E S I D
B L Y C L O S A A I S N N L C T U E D N A O T C
E P N O M D N L A E U O L T E E M S D E B T E A C
T C N T I I U U A M A O N A D A T U U E L L I Y L
I A E C O S D R L Y E A P O D N C A E D I L V N O
O G I I D A L T U N F A V O R A B L E Y T A V G I
```

The IRB/IEC Knows It All

GCP 3.3.8

The investigator should promptly report the following to the Institutional Review Board/Ethics Committee (IRB/IEC): deviations from the protocol, changes of the protocol, changes increasing the risk to subjects and/or affecting significantly the conduct of the trial, all adverse drug reactions that are both serious and unexpected, new information that may adversely affect the safety of the subjects or the conduct of the trial. From the list of words below, search for all those that are reportable to the IRB according to GCP 3.3.8.

Drug overdose
Informed consent
Deviations
Adverse events
Visit reports
Serious AE
Study closure
Enrollment
Protocol updates
Advertisements

Did the Drug Cause the Reaction?

GCP 1.1

*(Find each **bolded** word in the word search below.)*

In the **preapproval** clinical **experience** with a new medicinal product or its new **usages**, particularly as the **therapeutic dose**(s) may not be established, all **noxious** and unintended **responses** to a medicinal product related to any dose should be considered **adverse drug reactions**. The phrase "responses to medicinal product" means that a **causal relationship** between a medicinal product and an adverse event is at least a **reasonable** possibility (i.e, the relationship cannot be ruled out). During an active clinical trial, investigators are expected to determine if the cause of the reaction is possible, probable, related, or not related.

```
E P I U R E A S I C R S B S A L A V D R N R N R H
O E T E O T V I S S O A D O C A O S O P E A A S R S
R E D V L U E A O R I P O T L A A C R P P T A U N O A S
E L O A S E E I I P C C N E S U S R R E B P O X E E A
B E E T A A A N L R C C E R P S E S R L L R N O P E A
U S R H G P U C S U G T A E A E S N E C B O A O G
S O D S E O S E P N A H E P L P T E I B D I P R A
A A A O D I D D S S S E P E I P U I V V E T O E U
B E L S D O C E E R U R L E B C P A O E O C B N O
L A L I E R E E G S O A O T L E H E R L D A S A N
E T D C T L T N U V I P A O E B R S G R E E U E L
N E H U A S T E A A X E A I D S A L G L S R S L C
C B E L E O L L R O U D S R A P N O N R G X U A
S B E E V E S O E N T E L B I S S O P E U G A E
P A R O E O L N X S I T P A U R P E S G R E B S
R L L T S D A E P P C A E S E S N R T A D A E E
R E I O O E I D L E P D L V R E E S B I E S E N A N
N E A N S G A I R S O E A R A O N O O E S R O O
E T P L P O L P A I E S R D X P S L T V B E R O E A
P T U N N L A S P E X E D O T R I S V E N E G P E
R L T U A A E D P N C R R E V D L U U A R V R E L
C U A O E A T G S C T A S S E U C L E S E S D B O A
E O P R O B A B L E R E E B N O L A E E A I A C
L S R R U L H B A I E O N I U S E T N A T G C P P
A T N P L S E I U O U S C V I A R E E S C E E S A
```

Going to the Source

GCP 1.52

*(Find each **bolded** word in the word search below.)*

Hospital records	**Photographs**
Clinical charts	**Microfilm**
Office charts	**Magnetic media**
Laboratory notes	**Xrays**
Diaries	**Subject files**
Checklists	**Nursing notes**
Pharmacy records	**Phone logs**
Microfiche	**Drug orders**

M S I S T O C L I N T I T L E G D B O S M R S L E
R R S R E D R O G U R D D N O L C E R G T O L M E H R
R C H S I I R S H P C L J H S S N R R F I T C O O
O R C O S D R R O C E R L A T I P S O H H E L E O A C D
E O C O T R L M S C P D R H C A R L E M O A N C D D
S S C P C A P L P H O T O G R A P H S M R C Y R C
M E S L M Y T O D T P H A R M A C C Y R E E C O R D S
N T I R I A M S D C I S H L C I C A O E I N O M S S
N O S R F N G P T Z O O X R F S M F C S M S T Y Y
G N S C H L I N T R S N H O M R F T O O O H A S D
I G N O O M A C E T C D R E C I O N O G C R R B S
A N T C I R M M I A T D C L N C T S X F L X O O E C
H I E F C S O T C T L I L A E E K P O G R P O B E E R
N S P O R R S P A M C C C D D C L H R C S D S A S O
D R M P E S U I L M S H M I A O C I X C O L L C R
G U H O R G B R S C A Y A E R P O P S S I I E I I
E N C D E T J C I R T R H R D O E S S T C L S E B
E A I F S A E H T R I C S A T I U R L O S N O O A
F G C A G S C S A E J A T A C S A N L H R L E M O
N I A T E N T M S L E I I L E S R F T R S E S S N
F S A I T E F H T K O E E G H I L A E O R H T R S
L E A C C O I E C S R E O R R E E A T N E G I I H
O O D S U N A L P R N C O S E C F I S I J C R R Y N
O C C S T A E E A C O R S G O L E N O H P L Y R D H Y
E C I A R P S I S O E H E D C C O G A I T L S S T R

The Meaning of a Serious Adverse Event (SAE)

GCP 1.50

(Find each bolded word in the word search below.)

A serious adverse event is any untoward medicinal **occurrence** that at any dose

- Results in **death**
- Is **life-threatening**
- Requires **inpatient hospitalization** or **prolongation** of existing hospitalization
- Results in **persistent** or **significant disability/incapacity** or
- Causes a **congenital anomaly/birth defect.**

Protocol Basics

GCP 6.0

(Search for the names of the topics generally included in a trial protocol according to GCP Section 6.0.)

General information	Quality control
Trial objective	Quality assurance
Trial purpose	Ethics
Trial design	Data handling
Subject selection	Recordkeeping
Subject withdrawal	Financing
Treatment of subjects	Insurance
Efficacy	Publication policy
Safety	Supplements
Statistics	

A M Y C I L O P N O I T A C I L B U P T A S G E R
E N I Q P P A Y S C I T S I T A S Q L U L R I I
I T T E A T O E C N A R U S N I A E P N T N I
N C S U G C I C A N I O C T P J Y E P E L P I T T
T S N N Z A T O F G C H N C B E T L N S N H F R O
A U T J I E I I N I L R T N W U E A T O I G U I C
C L E L U N G T S T I P E R M E T S P K A G A E E
A I N Y D A L T M E J S S P E D I U S R T O P L Z N
C C U C N L R U C D R O R Z N O E E T U O S W O R
S H A C A B S N R A L E L T E P A R R D P M S C B W
L I I L H O A R S A I S C C G F O P L S L L C P J A
A N O Y A A E N O I T A M R O F N I L A R R E N E G
G R R B T T S I O R C V A T S R I L I I R N I C D D
C C M C A A I S D T O U T N C R E C E R T L S T U
Q T O K D K T B I L L L Q T T A S V A T A A T I B
S N S B B N T D J O I E Y P D Y A M N C C Q S V A
N O I T C E L L E S T C E J B U S A T E T Y C R E L
R A H I I T J E S A F E T Y O E T S N J I E J F S
W I A A S A P S J Q U A L I T Y C O N T R O L S A
E T Q U A L I T Y A S S U R A N C E C Q O B S S J
E F O T A C T R E A T M E N T O F S U B J E C T S
A J S R R C C G S P N E A I M E A V T A I C T N R T
D E S U B J E C T W I T H D R A W A L E R E I A E
R R Y T L D E F E S T I N N Q O E I J J C M I I I H P
R E C O O R D K E E P I N G J C A T A O Y T R C F C

Warning: Prompt Action Required!

GCP 5.20

*(Find each **bolded** word in the word search below.)*

Noncompliance with the protocol, SOPs, GCP, and/or applicable **regulatory requirement**(s) by an investigator/**institution**, or by member(s) of the sponsor's staff should lead to **prompt action** by the sponsor to secure compliance. If the monitor and/or **auditor identify** serious and/or **persistent** noncompliance on the part of an investigator/institution, the **sponsor** should **terminate** the investigator's/institution's **participation** in the trial. When an investigator's/institution's participation is terminated because of noncompliance, the sponsor should **notify** promptly the regulatory **authority**(ies).

T L I M S T I T C O R Y P P T I Y T N Y N E R I O
O Y F L M O R O R Y T N M I R P T E E O U O T N A
E Y S N O R I R I O I T P N T C P I R F C N M P
Q R I A S I E S R C N O T N O N C T O R S N N N
R I A R O T N O T I F Y O I A I R Q I S I I S N R
T A S N P U H R T I M S O I N L I E M D L P C E E
T C I I Y T S E I T P I L S R U R R O T E P G O E
P T A A U I T P O U I P T S Y O N A O Y O U P A R E
O R I A E N E A E T M I I Y T O R I R N L T E E E
I R I I E R O O O T T I E P A A M F A F T R I Q
O I I U P O R S C U N U P I T N O I T C A T A F U
P S I O C T T N T A E R N O T O I O P P G N N U I
E P N E A P O I I T N T O O A T R T I I O M P F R
R Y I I U N O R I C R I N I T S Y T S P T F O F Y E
F I F I N N I P D C E M T E N I P M M E A M O M
T N E T S I S R E P S O A O N I M N T L P M Y N E
R P T E G N O O N I L T P R T R O I N Q O N C N N
P R O R M E C S T N R S I O T E R M I N A T E T T
M G H O T F N I O N N C M Y C P A I N A C A N O
N E R O R U T O F O S C I F S O T R E N A U I R
O M C P I I T P Y U T E T R O S P N A S R T M N N
O P T L C D S Y O R P R N O T N O N F A O E A N
Q T I Y R T R I A I T I A I T O N O N N E P R S
A S C U C T Y I A U T A P T C R R I R E Y O E N R
M T R S Q R I C E A N A S A N T O I E N O L R I I

Drug Facts
GCP 7.1

The Investigator Brochure (IB) is a compilation of the clinical and non-clinical data on the investigational product(s) that are relevant to the study of the product(s) in human subjects. Its purpose is to provide the investigators and others involved in the trial with the facts and information needed to facilitate their understanding of the rationale for, and their compliance with, many key features of the protocol. The GCP guideline 7.1 delineates the minimum information that should be included in an IB. Can you find some of the minimum contents of an IB in the word search below?

Title page

Pharmacology

Confidentiality

Dosages

Table of contents

Human effects

Summary

Data and guidance

Introduction

Marketing experience

Properties

Formulation

Nonclinical studies

Toxicology

Safety

Efficacy

Pharmacokinetics

Is the Site Qualified?

According to section 5.6 of the GCP guidelines, the sponsor is responsible for selecting the investigator(s)/institution(s). Each investigator should be qualified by training and expertise and should have adequate resources to conduct the trial for which the investigator is selected. Can you find names of the different evaluation tools that a sponsor may use to help assess the qualifications of an investigative site?

Availability	**Competing trials**
Ethics board	**Patient population**
Budget	**Curriculum vitae**
Pharmacy	**Staff experience**
Checklist	**Audits**
Laboratory	**Blacklists**
Accreditation	**Site tour**

S L B Y I L N G E I K I D T O L R R B C G T E E
R S E I L S E U B I K R A S S Y A Y T B C I E E T R
E B C E A O B S L A I R T G N I T E P M O C H E Y
S I I G S T P R A O O L E T S A K T I O T S
P T D I S O Y O P K I T T D A Y A E Y T C E A L O
I E L K L R E H D A Y P I L M I R T S U L D U M
R Y Y O M Z H I I P A B N S P T C O B O H I E I H
B I I T L O M A S I M A S L L H L O T E U T L I T
E E T C A R I A I E A C R O A A L A T D A O R I R T
C A P M P T D A C T U R I I R R O R C T R I I E A
N C D T E A C Y H D R D T U D I I R M D L O I O I
E C R C A L R I E R R N I C A N E T U A C C E B E B
I R K T U Y A C R I T A T H V P S B O C L O A T
R E C A K P N T K P C O E I S A I X A E P Y L U L
E D U N C O N X L A U A T C A Y P A T C A C T B E
P I D A P P B O I D L Y A P L R C C O B F U T S T O
X T L C B T A R S L U L L U C F T G R S U B S P R
E A R C U N C E T C M S T T A U S T P P A I N T P
F T C I D E I L N E V P T B R A E L D U L U A L P
F I L B G I E U A E I I A D L C I R V T E K S E N
A O T E E T I L R L T E D Y T I L I B A L I A V A
T N R T T A T L R I A M N U P I A L A P T R O R S
S U L I E P L S M R E E B E P T I A I E S S T C S
V E M A R S A C R U M E N L C C O D S U A P A T A T
B B A S S T S I L K C A L B B K N R U R I A R A T

Extra! Extra! Read All About It!

During a routine monitoring visit, the CRA found that the site enrolled three subjects onto a study before giving informed consent. One of the three subjects did not meet the study's inclusion/exclusion criteria. The subject screening logs, enrollment logs, and CRFs had not been completed by the study coordinator prior to the monitoring visit. Study drug administration records were incomplete. The site's pharmacist had a family emergency for which she had to leave the site early before meeting with the CRA. None of the laboratories used by the patient were listed on the Form 1572. The principal investigator was unavailable to meet with the CRA during the first part of the visit, and left for home during the latter part of the visit. According to GCP Section 5.18.6, what should be included in the CRA's monitoring report after this visit?

Actions

Conclusions

Deficiencies

Deviations

Facts

Findings

Follow-up

Investigator name

Monitor name

Recommendations

Site

Site address

Summary

Visit date

Bonus Trivia Word Search

(Find the answers to these questions in the word search below.)

1) Prior to initiating a trial, the sponsor should _____, _____, and _____ all trial-related duties and functions. (GCP 5.7)

2) Neither the _____, nor the trial staff, should _____ or unduly influence a subject to participate or to continue to participate in a trial. (GCP 4.8.3)

3) Prior to a subject's participation in the trial, the written _____ form should be _____ and personally _____ by the _____ or by the subject's legally acceptable representative, and by the person who _____ the informed consent discussion. (GCP 4.8.8)

4) At the completion or termination of a trial, the following two reports should be filed at the site and with the sponsor: _____ and _____. (GCP 8.4)

5) In accordance with the sponsor's requirements, who is responsible for verifying that the investigator is enrolling only eligible subjects and that source documents and other trial records are accurate, complete, kept up-to-date, and maintained? _____ (GCP 5.18.4)

Copy That!

GCP 1.63 (addendum)

If original source documents cannot be accessed during a monitoring visit, then certified copies (irrespective of the type of media used) of the original records should be provided. *Take a few minutes from your busy day to find the words that describe the requirements for certified copies: **verified, signature, generation, identical, data, context, content, structure, original, media, copy, information***

O T X G N N M E O A I S O G I
T I Y I N T Y R F I I R I E O
R U E I M S P C M G T O N N O
G R F N R I O E N G T O F E T
L E G M N I C A S E O S O R T
N T N N S T T T E E T R A N
N I G I N U T I R D R T M T E
R D F N R I E T U T N T A I V
X E A E N I R M C E S E T O E
C N T T N T X E T N O C I N R
G T R M A R R N U T E I O T I
A I D E M D O A R O N U N T F
L C T S F C V R E I O O M R I
L A N I G I R O O L R O F N E
A L E C C E R O O T N T L E D

Is the Computer System Validated?

GCP 1.65 (addendum)

I am not a computer expert. Whenever asked to confirm if a computer system is validated, I request a statement from the institution's IT department to check if it mentions any of the below words which are relevant to GCP 1.65 and FDA's guidance for computerized systems used for data in clinical trials.

Enduring, lifecycle, operational, vendor, performance, design, backup, recovery, contingency, software, versions, dependability, security, signatures, maintenance, validated

Experience x Training = Qualifications

GCP 4.2.5 and 4.2.6 (addendum)

Qualifications are a product of experience and training. In clinical trials, the *investigator* is *responsible* for *supervising* any individual or party to whom the investigator *delegates* trial-related duties and *functions* conducted at the trial site. If the investigator/institution hires an independent party or individual to perform trial-related duties and functions, the investigator/*institution* should ensure this individual or party is *qualified* to *perform* those trial-related duties and functions and should *implement* procedures to ensure the *integrity* of the trial-related duties and functions performed and any data *generated*. Find the bolded words in the puzzle.

R O E L G N S B M I M P L E R M E N T D A
P E R F O R M U T I N S I N R T E I E G
G S L I O S B P A O E U E D T F T Q U G
N M E B B O V S E E S S T S S I E I E
S S P S G S I I F P R P G L R I F L P N
S I N T E G R I T Y O V S I E I I E I E
M N R U G E A S S U D C S E I T S E I
I S E D F S E I I E N E S R I U R T R
E T I F E F B T T G C I N G R V N R V A O
I I L V N L I Q E R T F I U E E G G R E
P T I N E V E L O P I I M T E I E N E E
L U T N T S L G I E O L E T N S T O N N
L T S O L A L I A I N A R A E T O I E D
U I O S I R T S E T S U S E R T I I G T
L O E N I G T S T E E Q T E F U G I E E
T N D N N E G T E N R N S R E E T O A Y S
A N F N E I O E T M S I I F C R S I D S
A I M A L O G R E T O N S E O I L N T E O
L R O T A G I T S E V N I E U O E S E I

ALCOA - C

GCP 4.9.0 (addendum)

In the 1990s, the acronym ALCOA was devised by Stan W. Woollen, a program coordinator in the FDA's Office of Enforcement for Bioresearch Monitoring (BIMO). ALCOA describes the fundamental principle of source documents being attributable, legible, contemporaneous, original, and accurate. In 2016, The International Council for Harmonization (ICH) E6(R2) addendum for Good Clinical Practices further added the "Complete"(C) principle to ALCOA. Named below are list of source documents/records in which ALCOA-C can be applied to.

Xrays	*Memoranda*	*Diaries*
Medical	*Consents*	*Obituary*
Nursing	*Laboratory*	*Pharmacy*
Questionnaires	*Echocardiogram*	*Diagnostics*

Risks Come with the Territory
GCP 5.0 (addendum)

Per ICH-GCP, the sponsor should decide which risks to reduce and/or which risks to accept. The approach used to reduce risk to an acceptable level should be proportionate to the significance of the risk. This puzzle contains a list of activities in which risk reductions may be incorporated a clinical trial. Can you find all of them?

study design
statistics
agreements
quality
communication

tolerance limits
project plans
deviations
SOPs
risk review

monitoring plans
safety
contracts
training

R Y S T N E M E E R G A I L A Y T E O O
A T C J O T O E E D D Y T O C C J I D C M
K A O R O K N N S T A T I S T I C S A I
N D M V I T Y V I A E T E A T N I I M A M
R N M M O S C S E T C E S F E M T I S A
T N U O S T K T Y V C S R K A R P N L U
S I N N A I Y R E E S C S P A S S E I G
R N I I G M S M S E R R Z E I D C M F T S
I A C T J I T C V S T N C P R P E S I
M N A O N L S P O S I I N E S R J M Z O
O L T R C E T E G M N E A I O L N J P O
M C I I Y C C P D G E E W J S O T T V O
L P O N S N A A T Y T S E N I C M S T Q
I S N G E A R A T E D C G V O N S O A J
T R P J R T L C J T J J G A I M M I E A
T Q E L O E N S E P I N T L S R A T A L
E A A G L O S L J J I I S D O R S N I
I D G N N O C A M N S N S S S L Y O C T
E S O S R T N G D E V I A T I O N S L Y
I S R P T S C R Q S N I E E N T I T N M

The Secret to Getting Clean Results

GCP 5.5.3 (a and b addendum)

Here lists the secret to getting clean results when using electronic trial data handling and/or remote electronic trial data systems. The sponsor should ensure:

completeness, accuracy, reliability, validation, functionality, maintenance, security, control, back-up, recovery, contingency, decommissioning, training, testing, SOPs

From Lemons 2 Lemonade: The Tale of Thalidomide

GCP 5.18.3 (addendum)

Beginning in 1959, the drug thalidomide[1,2] was found to cause disabilities in babies born to women who used it to treat morning sickness, and eventually banned in many countries; however, it was later found effective in treating and increasing the life span of patients diagnosed with multiple myeloma. Wow, let's talk about turning lemons into lemonade! In this brief historical look at thalidomide, we see how a drug with a negative outcome in one disease setting was found to have a positive outcome in a different disease setting after further tests were done on its mechanism of actions in humans. In clinical trials, developing and conducting safe studies are critical components for testing new drugs on humans. The addendum for GCP 5.18.3 outlines the considerations sponsors should make when planning their clinical trials. You'll find some of the words from these considerations in the puzzle below.

objective, on-site, systematic, prioritized, risk-based, centralized, remote, report, management, oversight, plan, visits

[1] Information from the Guardian online US edition, thalidomide Scandal: 60 year timeline, Press Association, Sep 1, 2012

[2] Licht J.D., Shortt I., and Johnstone R. (2014). *Cancer Cell, Vol. 25, Issue 1, p9-11, Jan. 13, 2014.*

```
A N A K T D G E I N A T R I A S A N T I E T L C T
J T E C C E N T R A L I N E D G S I D A N T T I P
H N T E C L N A I R R S M N S T H E T D O V R G
O S R O L M E C P E I V O E T E R E T N O A E E
S E E S M H I A M S P R V T I L S E E T N I L G N G
E O P R A G E O A S O P E P A O V E E T O R I S
H C O A M Y T A B R N P R N S R P A N E A T R R L
S O R E V E N B I A P S E M O M E M E T I T L
N E T E D O S I I M N T I T I T M E T E J T V A
T O R M S I D Z M R E I G I D V C I N I L T I V N
P T E R I L H L I E S O H P E I T E A E A N T E T
T E N N P R T S V G R B T O D A M V E E G A N T V
I P E T R E E M T R S T E E P E E V I T C E J B O D
E N T R I E E B E A D T E Y G R E S I I M D A M E
E B P T V A S P I A H D P L A Z M A I S V R O L A S
S V E A R E E O E M P R N D Z S I T Z E L A P E A
M I D R E Y I P A O I A C G Z E T S O A T V Z I B
O Z Z R I E V P P L M R Z T H D I I Z E I L V O K
I M A J M E M I R R T Z V C A T E R I R I A A S S
S Z E S Z A T E Z R M E I O R R E T C Z T O Z S I
T Z Z T Z O B S L Z E S Y S T E M A T I C P E V R
T T P T V S I M O T T D S A O I E V V I I E M I Z
E D I P H Z Y T K B D E Z I T I R O I R P E I P M
T A S K I E E T T G B O E H I E L E I I I O E T T
R Z Z A E E R C S I O Z C T K M G O E A S L M E C
```

Is Perfection a Reality?
GCP 5.20.1 (Addendum)

Find each bolded word.

I wish I knew of a clinical trial with no *mistakes*. I strove for *perfection* in the trials I *monitored* and *managed*, however, things always happened that *deviated* from the sponsor's *protocol* beyond anyone's *control* (ie. a subject's illness, electronic/ technical issues, missed appoints, human error, etc.). *Noncompliance* with the protocol, SOPs, GCP, and/or applicable *regulatory* requirement(s) by an investigator/institution, or by member(s) of the sponsor's staff should lead to *prompt* action by the sponsor to secure compliance. If noncompliance occurs that significantly affects or has the potential to significantly affect human subject *protection* or *reliability* of trial results, the sponsor should perform a *root-cause* analysis and implement appropriate *corrective* and *preventive actions*.

A D I V E E L O R T N O C R O I L A C P R R T L P
L T E I S I E E R V E E V C V O O M O G A P R E
O N E O E R E P T V A S A I T L V A O R T T O R N
O O N K S M O N P E M I J O T T S D N E C T D P O
O R Y I D A O A O E O A R A C A V T I F O A N T A
R J O E E N C A E T D L Y T G O V E T C J A E E C
A P N I N A C R T P C E O T C O E O A N T Y V E
I S S F P G C I E O R N P F R T E L R C M E T V O
I C O R R E C T I V E O O M V A A E I J L I D T
D N A C I D O N P I V J T C Y R T T D M O I L E P
N A V C I T O O T O E O V R L G I L I P I V I D E
O R T E A R E N N C N C N C O I D O S R E C B E N
O E O A G N M C S C T N O A E N O L I O S R A V I
E I D J E T R O E N I O C T L O O R T T J N I I I
A C S P T S I M O L V S Y O I N S N B E A K L A E
O S D E O O T P T E E I S T R L R C C O E T O
L C I R R D O S L N L C C E N N L N C T T T R E A
O O T R R I L I R I E T K N T E E R C I O E C D I
O I V D L D I A V N O O A T R K T D J O O R L O E
E P I L C J M N E E R T T R E O C C N R E I E R
T E R I V P I C E O C R S T I V N T N L C L L Y T
R N P N E R P E A T A O I K O C I V C L I F E E E
I P V O N C C O T S D I M T P E E M J C Y E K T
P O N B O O A C N E P A S T C T M O E O L G E N
P E R F E C T I O N E O E O E T C D R C M B M V

Location, Location, Location

GCP 8.1 (Addendum)

Be very, very careful; we are hunting in the puzzle below for hidden key words that describe who should maintain a record of location for essential documents, and how they should record them.

Bonus Trivia Word Search

(Find the answers to these questions in the word search below.)

1) Prior to initiating a trial, the sponsor should _____, _____, and _____ all trial-related duties and functions. (GCP 5.7)

2) Neither the _____, nor the trial staff, should _____ or unduly influence a subject to participate or to continue to participate in a trial. (GCP 4.8.3)

3) Prior to a subject's participation in the trial, the written _____ form should be _____ and personally _____ by the _____ or by the subject's legally acceptable representative, and by the person who _____ the informed consent discussion. (GCP 4.8.8)

4) At the completion or termination of a trial, the following two reports should be filed at the site and with the sponsor: _____ and _____. (GCP 8.4)

5) In accordance with the sponsor's requirements, who is responsible for verifying that the investigator is enrolling only eligible subjects and that source documents and other trial records are accurate, complete, kept up-to-date, and maintained? _____ (GCP 5.18.4)

FLASH CARDS

Instructions: Photocopy the following pages and cut them to use as travel size flash cards. The answers are located at the end of the flash cards section.

Question #1:

What is the difference between an Adverse Drug Reaction (ADR) and Adverse Event (AE) in the preapproval clinical experience with a new medicinal product or its usages?

Question #2:

According to *GCP section 8.2.4*, what document should be located in both the sponsor and investigator files before the Clinical Phase of the Trial formally starts?

Question #3:

Who is responsible for assuring that data submitted in an NDA is accurate and complete?

Question #4:

Clinical Trials should be conducted in accordance with the ethical principles that have their origin in what document?

Question #5:

A trial should be initiated and continued only if the anticipated benefits justify the risks. True or false?

Question #6:

How many days does a sponsor have to report a fatal or life threatening unexpected ADR to regulatory agencies after first knowledge that a case qualifies?

Question #7:

Who is responsible for safeguarding the rights, safety, and well-being of all trial subjects?

Question #8:

How many days does a sponsor have to report a serious, unexpected reaction that is not fatal or life threatening to the regulatory authorities after knowledge that a case qualifies?

Question #9:

Who is responsible for making the investigator selection?

Question #10:

While conducting a routine monitoring visit, the Clinical Research Associate discovered that a Serious Adverse Event (SAE) had not been reported to the Sponsor and IRB. What section of the ICH-GCP guidelines describes how the SAE should have been reported?

Question #11:

Data reported on the CRF are derived from shadow charts. True or false.

Question #12:

The principal investigator's education, training, and experience are referenced in what document described in GCP section 8.2.10?

Question #13:

Who should ensure the accuracy, completeness, legibility, and timelines of the data reported to the sponsor in the CRFs and all required reports? *(Guideline 4.9.1)*

Question #14:

What section of the GCP guidelines describes manufacturing, packaging, labeling, and coding of investigational products?

Question #15:

What does ICH stand for?

Question #16:

Before the clinical phase of a trial commences, a signed protocol and amendments are filed with the investigator/institution and sponsor. True or false?

Question #17:

What type of committee may a sponsor consider establishing to assess the progress of a clinical trial, including safety data and the critical efficacy endpoints at intervals, and to recommend to the sponsor whether to continue, modify, or stop a trial?

FLASH CARDS ANSWERS

Answer #1:
An ADR is any **harmful** or **unexpected** health response that is **related** to a medicinal (investigational) product.

An AE is any health occurrence, **expected** or **unexpected**, that occurs while a patient is participating on a clinical investigation trial, **whether** or **not** related to the investigational product. *(GCP 1.2 and 1.2)*

Answer #2:
Financial aspects of the trial: 1) A Clinical Study Agreement and 2) Financial Disclosure Forms.

Answer #3:
The sponsor *(GCP Section 5.1)*

Answer #4:
The Declaration of Helsinki *(GCP Section 2.1)*

Answer #5:
True. *(GCP Section 2.2)*

Answer #6:
Seven. *(Standard III B.1 of Clinical Safety Data Management)*

Answer #7:
The Institution Review Board *(GCP section 3.1.1)*

Answer #8:
Fifteen. *(Standard III B.2 of Clinical Safety Data Management)*

Answer #9:
The sponsor *(GCP Section 5.6)*

Answer #10:
Section 4.11

Answer #11:
False. Data reported on the CRF are derived from source documents (original documents, data, and records).

Answer #12:
Curriculum Vitae

Answer #13:
The investigator

Answer #14:
Section 5.13

Answer #15:
International Council for Harmonisation of technical requirements for registration of pharmaceuticals for human use

Answer #16:
True. (*GCP Section 8.2*)

Answer #17:
An Independent Data Monitoring Committee (IDMC) (*Guideline 5.5.2*)

REFERENCES

Dukett I (2005). *Learning styles: A perspective.* Learning and Skills Development Agency.

ICH Guidelines for Good Clinical as adopted by the FDA—Good Clinical Practice (E6), May 9, 1997, U. S. Federal Register, vol. 62.

International Council for Harmonisation (ICH) – ICH Harmonised Guideline, E6(R2) Good Clinical Practice: Integrated Addendum to E6(R1), Current Step 4 version, November 9, 2016, https://www.ich.org/page/efficacy-guidelines.

International Council for Harmonisation (ICH) – ICH Harmonised Guideline, General Considerations for Clinical Studies, Final Version, Adopted October 6, 2021, https://www.ich.org/page/efficacy-guidelines.

Rose C (1998). *Accelerated learning for the 21st century: The six-step plan to unlock your master-mind.* Bantam Doubleday Dell.

Smith A (1998). *Accelerated learning in practice: Brain-based methods for accelerating motivation and achievement.* (2003, 4th reprint). Network Educational Press Ltd.

WORD SEARCH SOLUTIONS

Solar Biomedical

Safety Is the Name of the Game

Solution

Find each bolded word in the word search below.

```
Q S A R O N I E A R N G T I D E P D E I G O N D G
N R I R I G H T S V N T N E A L Y G T E C T L I I
D G L L N D T I N C O R A I T P R I N C I P L E S
A G N I T C U D N O C A N S D S O I I I L R R O I
N E N G E E L I I L L A H I C R Q U A L I T Y I N
I O P A R T I C I P A T I O N N O E D I R G O I C
R T I S N A R T T G R R S P I I O C R E D I B L E
N C S N A R I T T N A S T O V A L P E N E R E Y T
E I Y F T N G H N I I T R R L G N O T R O G R I I
R R T Q I S G O N T T A R T R R Q S S I T Q E I L
I P E I O N A I R R N N O S I I C N C S C L A C S
I R F E N E A O T O T D L D O T L A O I I S L V C
D L A A A I P C D P Q A N I O S O N R R A A N S E
A L S P L L O C C E I R C I S D R D N C T I L A H
R H C R C C I V C R D I T N G N O O T V N V I D
B C E L T E C C T A F T C P I U T N S Y I R T E
E O I A I S C I E N T I F I C A S E I A C C S R G
V C E C L I N I C A L Y L T R N T R V D A I C R P
R G P R O T E C T E D R D A S H E N G P G D A N T
C I P I P O N V A C O C C O I C I P N L P I C T
O P C U R C I I C O A N C C T D U C I T V C E R S
E N N I N G A R S O T R A E R P Y N D L C A E E T
E S G E I I C R R N I L P T C L G C O I R P O T A
L I N V O L V E E E I P I A N I L R I N E S T G R
N N G A I N S C S C N E E F V O E C A G E T H I T
```

Words List

clinical	practice	international	ethical
scientific	quality	standard	designing
conducting	recording	reporting	trials
involve	participation	rights	safety
protected	principles	origin	credible

Can I Ever Throw Away Essential Documents?

Solution

(Find each bolded word in the word search below.)

```
O U D N M Y N A N I D M E E S Y I P R T E E K I A
I P Q C G I E S K T I S S E N E I P L P Y R A S D
N L P O D S I D A T S S A R A L I S A L M M G I G
E K G N S E R H R D E S M A A R B G C C E C E C L
N N R T T Y I N K N E P E I E E Y E M S R C D E I
E C G E R T Q U T L C E P E Q P Y N S T E L I C U
P A T M A S E I S D T I N N R R C S R Q N M C A
N E D P A R A P P L I C A T I O N A T E N E N M A
I I E L T L U R T P U S L R I S R L M S R A E S M
I T N A C L A G R E E M E N T G L R O P N R M I U
P I I T Q I T I M B E E G N E C O E U O E E E T E
D U A E A E E E S M T S E M N G S Q C N N N S E O
S T T D L M L L K T E M A L S I I U M S P I D E E
M R E T P E M P M L U R C T P I D I S I S S S L C
I E R P E U T D T C K L O E E E R R N B Y E B C R
N E Y O I A L E O E M C M I C H R E G I O N C T L
I E P I E R I D T I E E N I R S M M I L G N P O S
E T S N M R N I A D N E S E I O L E C I O P A I E
D E Y K T C N E I D I R M M E N L N S T L S S L R
U A S S P G O B H R T I N T I T I T C Y E Y D A E
E A E U A M R S T D P Q R I L A Y S I E D G I U N
N T R E T E E Q C R D S A E L A P S E D G N A G M
A S N O R N E R B E E O I A T I T T E S K I M E S
S R T P N T E I S Y E I D E O T T L E I E M G E E
E E N L N S R D Y N I S N E P G P I M I L O K I M
```

Words List

AGREEMENT	APPLICATION	CONTEMPLATED	ELAPSED
ESSENTIAL	DOCUMENTS	ICHREGION	MARKETING
REQUIREMENTS	RESPONSIBILITY	RETAINED	YEARS

Names of Documents Found in Both the 21 CFRs for Clinical Research and the ICH/GCP Guidelines

Solution

(Find each word in the word search below.)

```
T C A T M E T E R N V P O S E S P P R T E O M R R E
C L P I O Y O O D T E S T O P E R S P R U L O U T T
U P R P T R A R T R I R S I U L T P I C S P R R P N
R X A R R N A T T A T R S P T R S A T N M O E R P C
E L U L O A G M R S O X R T A T I T R E U L O R E U
O E E T P P D A R T S E N T N D D X O O P S T S M R
O A P M E O E R U R O S S E R E R S P P T X U N R R
S R V T R X U E L E T P M R M R D C E R A E E E T I
H P S I D E I T E U B D Y P G X U D R O E M E E I C
I R F N E F T P R T N I C R I U M L Y G P R R U R U
P P P R T U S P S E A A R R O F P T T R M E D R S L
P M R P I E R R M P G L R N N M R N E E R U O D E U
I T F S D P A A E R S A A R R M O S F S S T R E S M
N S G R E E E T R O P E R L A U N N A S R E R O S V
G L D A P O R R L T O P R O D N R S S R O P U M N I
R A A S X A D R T O R C O P R T I E T E R N S D P T
E V L L E D U U R C N T O S D R P P N P R M A P L A
C O E C P P R C E O A E C P V O E P R O O D L R S E
O R A R E V T F U L M R O F T R O P E R E S A C N A
R P R G O E S E P S E B O E A A P E R T I S C T I C
D P P D O F R C U S O S E A E N M F V E P L E R S R
S A P L P R P T R P L T O A U L I I P X M R T T C E A
S B M P C R O S D T E F S S A P R D I R M T S P T E
E R R O M A U O R G O I L A D T A G C P O E T O E R
D I H P V G S T N E M U C O D E C R U O S S B N O L
U R E E O E R R E M R E R U P M F R R O E I I O C C
```

AMENDMENTS
ANNUALREPORT
CASEREPORTFORM
CURRICULUMVITAE
EXPEDITEDREPORT
IRBAPPROVALS
PROGRESSREPORT
PROTOCOLS
SAFETYREPORT
SHIPPINGRECORDS
SOURCEDOCUMENTS

Knowing the Signs and Symptoms

Solution

Find each bolded word in the word search below.

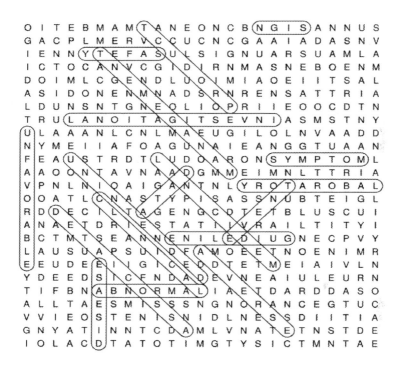

Words List

ABNORMAL	ADVERSE	ASSOCIATED	CLINICAL
DATA	DISEASE	EVENT	GUIDELINE
INVESTIGATIONAL	LABORATORY	MANAGEMENT	MEDICINAL
PRODUCT	SAFETY	SIGN	SYMPTOM
UNFAVORABLE	UNINTENDED		

The IRB/IEC Knows It All

Solution

From the list of words below, search for all those that are reportable to the IRB according to GCP 3.3.8

```
D C E E D D R S E E I L E R V V O A E C T T R O A
I E L T C S O O E E O E E D V O A O R O S O C E N
T T S E E I D I T E L S E A M L E E L I V R V T E
E N E V T R M T P N E V A G O S E V I S S N E V
I E V I E R E E O T I T N N T N A E N T D S T N A
E M P D R O O E E A E R P E N O O R C T R R O N D
R E E V E E A I T N E S N O C D E M R O F N I E U
N S M I V O T I N M R D L L E L L D T I U D O E
I I V S D R O D E E S O D R E V O G U R D U N O S
A T N I R N T A V P E U L E E V R E R E S C O S M
I R N O S E T S E L G T D L S E P O I R T O D A T
L E D P E O N R E V S N E T M R O E O E I A N E R
E V I S E N D T S O U D O E E E T L I L S C S A D
E D S T V O S C R S R O O E U R N D R C M T T S P
A A L R I E E D E V A S S T O I E T S P U R O U E
P C V O D D L E V O S I E P R E E E E D N D E O S
O E L S T T S S D E I R E P E V I T Y E R D O I P
R U S O S R E I A D O R V C E S R C E I C U A R E
R M D U T O E O U M T O S S V D L V S E S L V E A
E V T R O V N T E I T O S C D O T S G N D E E S U
T A P S P L D V S D T N N P S R O V P O U L I E D
E E O S P T U I E E O T U U E U V D V R I U N E S
E E U P A R V E F S C T R I N C N P O O I S E T N
P R T E S N T S C R I E T A D P U L O C O T O R P
R F R O D T E E T S E I M V D O S S E O I O V O C
```

Words List

Drugoverdose	Informedconsent	Deviations	adverseevent
visitreport	SeriousAE	Studyclosure	enrollment
Protocolupdate	Advertisement		

Did the Drug Cause the Reaction?

Solution

Find each bolded word in the word search below.

```
A  L  E  C  R  P  E  N  R  R  P  S  C  N  E  L  B  A  S  U  B  E  R  O  E
T  S  O  U  L  T  T  E  E  L  A  B  T  E  T  A  E  A  O  S  E  L  D  E  P
N  R  P  A  T  U  P  E  I  E  R  E  E  H  D  L  L  A  D  R  E  O  V  T  I
P  R  R  O  U  N  L  A  O  L  O  E  E  U  C  I  S  O  S  H  T  A  L  E  U
L  U  O  E  A  N  P  N  O  T  R  E  L  A  T  E  D  D  E  G  A  S  U  O  R
S  L  B  A  A  L  O  S  E  S  E  V  E  S  L  R  O  I  O  P  A  E  E  T  E
E  H  A  T  E  A  L  G  I  D  O  E  O  T  T  E  C  D  S  U  A  E  A  V  A
I  B  B  G  D  S  P  A  D  A  L  S  L  E  N  E  E  D  E  C  N  I  O  I  S
U  A  L  S  P  P  A  I  L  E  N  O  L  A  U  G  E  S  P  S  L  I  R  S  I
O  I  E  C  N  E  I  R  E  P  X  E  R  A  V  S  R  S  N  U  R  P  I  S  C
U  E  R  T  C  X  E  S  P  P  S  N  O  X  I  O  U  S  A  G  C  C  P  O  R
S  O  E  A  R  E  S  O  D  C  I  T  U  E  P  A  R  E  H  T  E  N  O  A  S
C  N  E  S  R  D  R  E  L  A  T  E  D  A  A  O  L  P  E  A  R  E  T  D  B
V  I  B  S  E  O  D  A  V  E  P  L  S  I  O  T  E  E  P  S  L  O  S
I  U  N  E  V  T  X  R  E  S  A  B  R  D  E  L  B  I  L  A  S  U  A  C  A
A  S  O  U  D  R  P  A  E  E  U  I  A  S  B  E  C  P  P  E  E  S  A  O  L
R  E  L  C  L  I  S  O  S  S  R  S  P  A  R  H  P  U  T  S  S  R  C  S  A
E  T  A  E  U  S  L  N  B  N  P  S  N  L  S  E  A  I  E  N  R  R  P  O  V
E  N  E  S  U  V  T  O  I  R  E  O  O  G  G  R  O  V  I  E  L  E  P  P  D
S  A  E  E  A  E  V  O  E  T  S  P  N  L  R  L  E  V  B  C  L  B  T  E  R
C  T  G  S  R  N  B  E  S  A  G  E  R  S  E  D  O  E  D  B  R  P  A  A  N
E  P  A  D  V  E  R  S  E  D  R  U  G  R  E  A  C  T  I  O  N  O  U  A  R
E  C  I  B  R  G  O  R  N  A  E  G  X  S  U  S  B  O  P  A  O  X  N  S  N
S  P  A  O  E  P  E  O  A  E  B  A  U  L  E  A  N  E  R  O  P  E  O  R  R
A  P  C  A  L  E  A  O  N  E  S  E  A  C  L  N  O  U  A  G  A  R  A  S  H
```

Words List

Preapproval	Experience	Usage	Therapeutic dose
Noxious	Responses	Adverse drug reaction	Causal
Reasonable	Probable	Possible	Related
Not related			

Going to the Source

Solution

Find each bolded word in the word search below.

```
E  O  O  L  F  N  F  E  E  G  D  N  H  A  I  G  N  N  M  S  E  O  R  R  M
C  C  D  E  S  I  G  A  N  U  R  S  I  N  G  N  O  T  E  S  O  R  C  S  S
I  S  S  A  A  A  C  I  C  H  M  P  F  T  N  S  S  I  S  C  C  O  H  R  I
A  T  U  A  I  T  A  F  D  O  P  O  C  C  O  C  R  R  L  P  O  S  S  E  S
R  A  N  C  T  E  G  S  E  R  E  R  S  I  O  H  F  I  M  C  T  D  I  D  T
P  E  A  O  E  N  S  A  T  G  S  R  O  R  M  L  N  A  Y  A  R  R  I  R  O
S  E  L  I  F  T  C  E  J  B  U  S  T  M  A  L  G  M  T  P  L  O  R  O  C
I  A  P  E  H  M  S  H  C  R  I  P  C  I  C  N  P  S  O  L  M  C  S  G  L
S  C  R  C  T  S  A  T  I  S  L  A  T  A  E  T  T  D  D  P  S  E  H  U  I
O  O  N  S  K  F  E  R  R  C  M  M  M  L  T  R  N  C  T  H  C  R  P  R  N
E  R  C  R  O  E  J  I  I  A  S  O  I  D  C  S  O  I  P  O  P  L  C  D  T
H  S  O  E  E  I  A  C  R  H  C  L  C  D  N  C  S  H  T  D  A  L  D  I
E  G  S  O  E  I  T  S  H  A  M  C  A  L  R  H  X  H  A  O  R  T  J  N  T
D  O  E  R  G  L  A  A  R  E  I  D  E  N  E  O  R  L  R  G  H  I  H  O  L
C  L  C  R  H  E  C  T  D  R  A  D  E  C  C  M  F  C  M  R  C  P  S  L  E
O  E  F  E  I  S  S  I  O  P  O  C  K  T  I  R  S  I  A  A  A  S  S  C  G
G  N  I  E  L  R  A  U  E  O  C  L  P  S  O  F  M  C  C  P  R  O  N  E  D
A  O  S  A  A  F  N  R  S  P  I  H  O  X  N  T  F  A  Y  H  L  H  R  G  B
I  H  I  T  E  T  L  L  S  S  X  R  G  F  O  O  C  O  R  S  E  H  R  T  O
T  P  J  N  O  R  H  O  T  S  C  S  R  L  G  O  S  E  E  M  M  E  F  O  S
L  Y  C  E  R  S  R  S  C  I  O  D  P  X  C  O  M  I  C  R  O  F  I  L  M
S  R  R  G  H  E  L  N  L  I  L  S  O  O  R  H  S  N  O  C  A  E  T  M  R
S  D  R  I  T  S  E  O  S  E  L  A  B  O  R  A  T  O  R  Y  N  O  T  E  S
T  H  Y  I  R  S  M  O  E  I  C  S  E  E  B  S  Y  M  D  R  C  A  C  H  L
R  Y  N  H  S  N  O  A  B  I  R  O  R  C  S  D  Y  S  S  C  D  C  O  R  E
```

Words List

Hospital records	Clinical charts	Office charts	Laboratory notes
Diaries	Checklists	Pharmacy records	Microfiche
Photographs	Microfilm	Magnetic media	Xrays
Subject files	Nursing notes	Phone logs	Drug orders

The Meaning of a Serious Adverse Event (SAE)

Solution

Find each bolded word in the word search below.

Words List

Hospital records	Clinical charts	Office charts	Laboratory notes
Diaries	Checklists	Pharmacy records	Microfiche
Photographs	Microfilm	Magnetic media	Xrays
Subject files	Nursing notes	Phone logs	Drug orders

Protocol Basics

Solution

Find each bolded word in the word search below.

R R D A E E W R N S Q C G A L S C A C A T N I E A
E T E J F T I A O N T C R N H C I L U S C T N M
C Y S S O Q A H I S O M R O I A U N M T N S T I Y
O T U R T U A I T B K C B Y L C C Y E J N U T Q C
R L B R A A S I C B D A T A H A N D L I N G E P I
D E J C C L A T E N K A T A O B L A U E A C A P L
K F E G T I P J L T T I S E A S R L N T I T A O
E S C S R T S E E D B S I N R N U T G I Q C O Y P
E T T P E Y J S S J I D O O S R C M T N F A E S N
P I W N A A Q A T O L T R I A L D E S I G N C C O
I N I E T S U F C I L O C T I E R J T L C I N I I
N N T A M S A E E E L U V A S L O S I R H O A T T
G Q H I E U L T J Y Q T A M O T R S P T N C R S A
J O D M N R I Y B P T N T R G E N P E N C T U I C
C E R E T A T O U D T C S O F P N E R W B P S T I
A I A A O N Y E S Y A R R F O A O D M U E J N A L
T U W V F C C T A A S E I N P R E I E E T Y I T B
A U A T S E O S T M V C L I L R E U T A L E A S U
O C L A U C N N E N A E I L S D T S S T N P E Q P
Y M E I B Q T J T C T R I A L P U R P O S E P L T
T I R C J O R I Y C A T R R L M O T K I N L N U A
R I E T E B O E C Q A L N E C S S O A G H P T L S
C I I N C S L U R S T S I N P C W P G U F I N R G
F H A R T S S F E V I T C E J B O L A I R T N I E
C P E T S J A S L A B U D G A W R N E C O T I I R

Words List

General information	Trial objective	Trial purpose	Trial design
Subject selection	Subject withdrawal	Treatment of subjects	Efficacy
Safety	Statistics	Quality control	Quality assurance
Ethics	Data handling	Recordkeeping	Financing
Insurance	Publication policy	Supplements	

Warning: Prompt Action Required!

Solution

Find each bolded word in the word search below.

```
M A Q O O N M P R T F R E P O I O P T T R Q E O T
T S T P M E G R M N T Y P S I R R T C A I R Y Y L
R C I T C R H O T E F I N I I I I A I S A I S F I
S U Y T P O O R E T I I E O U I A A I N R A N L M
Q C R L I R T M G S N U A C P E E U Y P O S O M S
R T T C I U T E N I N N P T O R N I T U T I T O T
I Y R D T T F C O S I O O T R O E T S H N E R R I
C I I S P O N S O R P R I N S O A P E R O S I O T
E A A Y Y F I T N E D I I T C O E O I T T R R R C
A U I O U O O N I P C R T A U O T U T I I C I Y O
N T T R T S N R L S E I N E N T M I P M F N O T R
A A I P E C N S T O M N T R U T P I S Y O I N Y
S P A R T I C I P A T I O N P I I T L O O T T M P
A T I N R F M O R O E T O O I E Y S S I N P I P
N C T O O S Y T T N N S A T T P T Y R N A O N R T
T R T T S O C E R I I Y T O N A O O U L N T P I
O R O N P T P R O M P T R I O A R N R I R C C T Y
I I N O N T A M I N M S T O I M I A R E Q T P E T
E R O N A R I I N T M P I P T F R O O M I O I E N
N E N F S E N N Q L M T I P C A N Y T D S R R O Y
O Y N A R N A A O P E F O G A F L O E L I S F U N
L O E O T A C T N M A O M N T T T U P P I N C O E
R E P E M U A E C Y M F P N A R E P G C S N N T R
I N R A N I N T N N O Y F U F I E A O E N N M N I
I R S N M R O T N E M E R I U Q E R E E R N P A O
```

Words List

Noncompliance	Regulatory	Requirement	Institution
Prompt	Action	Identify	Persistent
Sponsor	Terminate	Participation	Notify
Authority			

Drug Facts

Solution

```
C L Y G G D S D E I Y I A I U F B F D A U A A N S
P H A R M A C O L O G Y T A S O I C E A O T A S C
F A E E C D Y T I L A I T N E D I F N O C I E X I
K X I O U T M T K O I A S A R R F C D F T E X O T
G F O R M U L A T I O N A U A L I O E S I I D O E
O E E G U U C B N O D A P T I T I P A S O T A E N
U R P K E Y S L E O S N C D I H E E I U C T N A I
I I E T I T L E P A G E O I U F M I T M F I A A K
R O T O T E E O M E N T L M F O N Y I M T E A D O
S D K X E A A F A I C E A E R P C I A U E I A C
I O A I O P L C O S I N C S P R O P E R T I E S A
U S T C P S I O I N E A A G Y E N M L Y I E Y N M
G A H O O S O N S F C A C D P T P A O T A R O R R
L G I L P M C T F Y D N T A I E M T K O A C T I A
A E I O E D C E I M N H L A R U C F E M T P R E H
L S U G C E C N U E N A Y T T N G C C A N G Y E P
M S E Y G T D T A L R E N N N R D D P E O Y O S A
N O U T S R T S A N L P F R G D I N N R N Y I R E
E C N E I R E P X E G N I T E K R A M A S A O M P
E S L F N N O I T C U D O R T N I L A U A T P N A
T P O A L D C I C C T M S S A L E C F L R T R M C
N O T S A I O O T D D N R L S G R A I T N C A H U
U A A E F I T I I E Y G N A E D I M R S P A A D F
S E I D U T S L A C I N I L C N O N N N Y S N T M
A N L P D S F A C C O I N U H G N N I L Y O F O F
```

Words List

Title page	Pharmacology	Confidentiality	Dosages
Table of contents	Human effects	Summary	Data and guidance
Introduction	Marketing experience	Properties	Formulation
Nonclinical studies	Toxicology	Safety	Efficacy
Pharmacokinetics			

Is the Site Qualified?

Solution

```
B V S T A F F E X P E R I E N C E B R I P S E R S
B E U N O I T A T I D E R C C A T I Y E T I B S L
A M L R T L C R L D U C K R D P C I Y L D I C E B
S A I T E B I C C A N A T C T M A T O K I I E I Y
S R E T E G D U B P C K T A E P R L M L S G A L I
T S P A T I E N T P O P U L A T I O N R O S O S L
S A L T I E I C A B N N Y R C D A M H E Y T B E N
I C S L L U L E R O X T A I Y A I A I H O T S U G
L R M R R A N T S I L K C E H C E S I D P P L B E
K U R I L E E C L D A P R R D T A I P A K R A I I
C M E A T I V M U L U C I R R U C M A Y I I I K K
A N E M E I P S L Y A O T N D R R A B P T A R R I
L L B N D A T T L A T E A I T I O S N I T O T A D
B C E U Y D B T U P C I T C U I A L S L D O G S T
B C P P T F R A C F A S H A D R A L P M A L N S O
K O T I I C A U F R Y A V N I R H T I Y E I Y L
N D I A L I E S T C P I P E I O A L C R A T I A R
R S A L I R L T G C A X S T R R T O O T E S E Y R
U U I A B V D P R B T A B U M C D T B T Y A P T B
R A E P A T U P S F C E O A D T A E O S T K M B C
I P S T L E L A U U A P C C L R O U H U C T O I G
A A S R I K U I B T C Y L E O I R T I L E I C E T
R T T O A S A N S S T L O B I I I L E D A O H E E
A A C R V E L T P T B U A E O E R I I U L T E T E
T T S S A N P P R O E L T B I A T T H M O S Y R E
```

Words List

Availability	Ethics Board	Budget	Pharmacy
Checklist	Laboratory	Accreditation	Competing trials
Patient population	Curriculum vitae	Staff experience	Audits
Blacklists	Site tour		

Extra! Extra! Read All About It!

Solution

```
I N C E I S D M F D E N A T N U V I A D W F N E I
R E E M I S S C D R S A E N N N M I P I T T G M N
I O O D N I T N D T D A I I T A E C S E M S E R F
R C I E D F O V T S T D E A E E N N I I N E T M S
I T T A C S S D T S I D I S N N I I M N A A R L D
C N N C E E F U E I E F A N D N A E C N E L U F E
S T I I M U U I E O E C I L V T D E V N E I S S S
S T O F O A I C S I E A T E S R F O L L O W U P T
I N O N U S U W N S O C S S I I W D S T C E A A S
T D O Y D U E L S M I T E E N I E I T E T O N I N
E D N R T U S V E F I N D S E T A D T I S I V O
A E F A I R S M P G C O I O M I T A T C O D S I
D A T M M C S D A N U N A C M A S O I T G C O I T
D S D M N I T T E N G S A S N N T F E U D T I A A
R R T U I R O I M S S I S I D R F S D I T S S A D
E M T S C R C V S E E I G C S O T E O R T A S A N
S C T T N I N V E I I D C F U T V E I S A C P C E
S A M A F E T I N N M S E A T I M N S I S I A S M
T E M E U T M R N I T C S C A N D I F N M A C I M
I E D O S O C N G T E S D T Y O M C E N D N D O O
D O R I D L I N M I O U I S R M A C I E N T N O C
T E D O C S R A E A C O N C L U S I O N S F I L E
N I N T W T I N E N N G S E T F N R W I O R O V R
T O T C N V S T Q S S S O T O S S N T O O A I R R
U C N N A S V S E N A N N U N N T E G N L W E L S
```

Words List

Actions	Conclusions	Deficiencies	Deviations
Facts	Findings	Follow up	Investigator name
Monitor name	Recommendations	Site	Site address
Summary	Visit date		

Copy That!

Solution

GCP 1.63 (addendum)

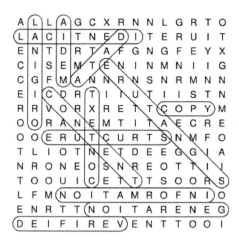

Words List

verified	signature	generation	identical
data	context	content	structure
original	media	copy	information

Is the Computer System Validated?

Solution

GCP 1.65 (addendum)

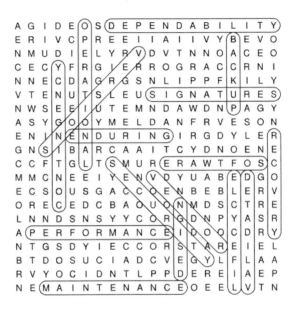

Words List

Enduring	lifecycle	operational	vendor
performance	design	backup	recovery
contingency	software	versions	dependability
security	signatures	maintenance	validated

Experience x Training = Qualifications

Solution

GCP 4.2.5 and 4.2.6 (addendum)

```
L  A  A  T  L  U  L  P  P  I  E  I  M  N  S  S  N  G  P  R
R  I  N  N  O  I  T  U  T  I  T  S  N  I  I  S  M  S  E  O
O  M  F  D  E  O  S  T  I  L  I  E  R  N  N  P  E  L  R  E
T  A  N  N  N  S  O  N  N  V  F  D  U  P  T  S  E  I  F  L
A  L  E  N  I  I  L  T  E  N  E  F  G  E  E  G  B  O  O  G
G  O  I  E  G  R  A  S  V  L  F  S  E  E  G  S  O  S  R  N
I  G  O  G  T  T  L  L  E  A  B  E  A  F  R  I  V  T  M  S
T  R  E  E  S  S  I  G  L  Q  T  I  S  S  I  I  S  B  U  B
S  E  T  N  T  E  A  I  O  E  T  I  S  R  T  F  E  P  T  M
E  O  M  R  E  T  I  E  P  R  G  E  U  N  Y  P  E  A  I  I
V  N  S  N  E  S  N  O  I  T  C  N  U  F  O  R  S  O  N  M
N  S  I  S  Q  U  A  L  I  F  I  E  D  T  V  P  S  E  S  P
I  E  I  R  T  S  R  E  M  I  N  S  C  I  S  G  S  U  I  L
E  O  F  E  E  E  A  T  T  U  G  R  S  P  I  L  T  E  N  E
U  I  C  E  F  R  E  N  E  E  V  I  E  S  E  R  S  D  R  M
O  L  R  T  U  T  T  S  I  E  N  I  I  O  I  I  S  T  T  E
E  N  S  O  G  I  O  T  E  G  R  U  T  C  I  F  I  F  E  N
S  T  I  A  I  I  I  O  N  G  V  R  S  I  E  L  E  T  I  T
E  E  D  Y  E  G  E  N  E  R  A  T  E  D  I  P  I  Q  E  D
I  O  S  S  E  T  D  N  E  E  O  R  I  G  E  N  E  U  G  A
```

Words List

investigator	responsible	supervising	delegates
functions	institution	qualified	perform
implement	integrity	generated	

ALCOA-C

Solution

GCP 4.9.0 (addendum)

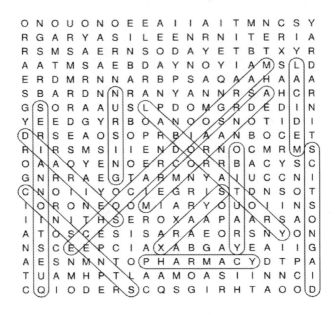

Words List

Xrays	Medical	Nursing	Questionnaires
Memoranda	Consents	Laboratory	Echocardiogram
Diaries	Obituary	Pharmacy	Diagnostics

Risks Come With the Territory

Solution

GCP 5.0 (addendum)

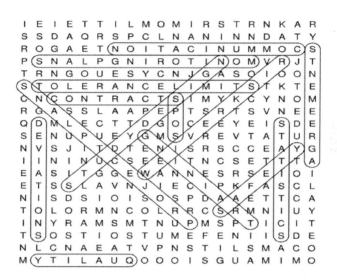

Words List

study design	tolerance limits	monitoring plans	statistics
project plans	safety	agreements	deviations
contracts	quality	SOPs	communication
training	risk review		

The Secret to Getting Clean Results

Solution

GCP 5.5.3 (a and b addendum)

Words List

completeness	accuracy	reliability	validation
functionality	maintenance	security	control
backup	recovery	contingency	decommissioning
training	testing	SOPs	

From Lemons 2 Lemonade: The Tale of Thalidomide

Solution

GCP 5.18.3 (addendum)

```
C T E T T S I O M S E E I T P T N S H E S O H J A
R A D T N N M N I V B N P E T O E O C O E S N T N
Z S I P N E A Z D E P T E N E R T R O P E R T E A
A K P T T S J R R A T R T N R M E E A R S O E C K
E I H V Z N M I E R V I E P I S D V M A M L T C T
E E N S O A E E Y E A E E R L I O E Y G H M L E D
R E Y I B T M V I E S E M T H D S E T E I E N N G
C T T M S E I P P O P B T S L Z I N A O A C A T E
S T K O L Z R P A E I E R V I M I B A A M P I R I
I G B T N R R L O M A A S G E R M I R S S E R A N
O B D T E M T M I P H D T R S E N A N O P R L A
N O E D S E N R A R P T E B O I T P P P R V S I T
C E Z S Y I V N C N L E E T H G I S R E V O M Z R
T H I A S O C T G D A Y P O P I T E N P T E N E I
K I T O T R A H N N N G E D E D I M S A I E S D A
M E I I E R T D E S M R E A I V T O R O L T T G S
G L R E M E E I T I A E V M T C T M P V S E H S A
O E O V A T R I S T I S I V E I M E A E E R T I N
E I I V T C I N O N S I T E A N E M N E T E E D T
A I R I I Z R E A E V I C E E T M E T N T T A I
S I P I C T I I I T L R M E G A L E E A O I N D N E
L O E E P O A L V A O D J A Z T J T T R L O O T T
M E I M E N A V N P L A B N T I T I R T G A V T L
E T P I V S S O I E A M O T E V V T R I N E R I C
C T M Z R I S K B A S E D V T N A L L S G E G P T
```

Words List

objective	onsite	systematic	prioritized
riskbased	centralized	remote	report
management	oversight	plan	visits

Is Perfection a Reality?

Solution

Find each bolded word.
GCP 5.20.1 (Addendum)

```
P  P  I  R  T  E  O  O  L  O  A  E  O  O  N  D  I  I  A  R  O  O  O  L  A
P  O  P  N  E  P  I  O  C  S  C  I  E  R  A  N  C  S  P  U  R  O  N  T  D
E  N  V  P  R  I  V  T  I  D  S  D  O  T  V  A  O  S  N  O  Y  N  E  T  I
R  B  O  N  I  L  D  R  R  E  P  U  A  E  C  C  R  F  I  E  I  K  O  E  V
F  O  N  E  V  C  L  R  D  O  T  E  G  A  I  I  R  P  N  E  D  S  E  I  E
E  O  C  R  P  U  D  I  O  O  S  T  N  R  T  D  E  G  A  N  A  M  R  S  E
C  A  C  P  I  M  I  L  S  T  I  R  M  E  O  O  C  C  C  C  O  O  E  I  L
T  C  O  E  C  N  A  I  L  P  M  O  C  N  O  N  T  I  R  A  A  N  P  E  O
I  N  T  A  E  E  V  R  N  T  O  E  S  N  T  P  I  E  T  E  O  P  T  E  R
O  E  S  T  O  E  N  I  L  E  L  N  C  C  O  I  V  O  T  T  E  E  V  R  T
N  E  D  A  C  R  O  E  C  E  V  I  T  N  E  V  E  R  P  D  O  M  A  V  N
E  P  I  O  R  T  O  T  C  I  S  O  N  C  O  U  O  N  C  L  A  I  S  E  O
O  A  M  I  S  T  A  K  E  S  Y  C  O  N  V  T  O  P  E  Y  R  U  A  E  C
E  S  T  K  T  R  T  N  N  T  O  T  A  C  R  C  M  F  O  T  A  O  I  V  R
O  T  P  O  I  E  R  T  N  R  I  L  E  O  L  Y  V  R  T  G  C  T  T  C  O
E  C  E  C  V  E  K  E  L  L  N  O  N  I  G  R  A  T  C  O  A  T  L  V  I
T  T  E  I  N  O  T  E  N  R  S  O  O  D  I  T  A  E  O  V  V  S  V  O  L
C  M  T  V  T  C  D  R  C  C  N  R  L  O  L  T  L  L  E  E  T  D  A  O  A
D  O  M  C  N  C  U  C  T  E  B  T  I  S  I  D  E  R  O  T  I  N  O  M  C
R  E  U  L  L  N  O  I  T  C  E  T  O  R  P  M  I  C  A  C  F  E  R  O  P
C  O  C  I  C  R  O  O  T  C  A  U  S  E  I  O  U  M  N  U  O  C  T  G  R
M  L  Y  F  L  E  R  E  T  O  K  N  R  C  V  I  L  E  T  A  A  T  A  R
B  G  E  E  L  I  L  C  R  E  L  I  A  B  I  L  I  T  Y  E  N  D  O  P  T
M  E  K  E  Y  E  O  D  E  T  A  I  V  E  D  E  D  V  V  E  T  P  R  R  L
V  N  T  E  T  R  E  I  A  O  E  I  I  N  E  P  T  O  E  C  A  O  N  E  P
```

Words List

mistakes	perfection	monitored	managed
deviated	protocol	control	noncompliance
rootcause	protection	reliability	corrective
preventive			

Location, Location, Location

Solution

GCP 8.1 (Addendum)

```
C R E C O R D R I U E R M V G T I L T N O N O N R
I I O C A D R R H O I E R E L N I L S R R E V L I
T C C A N N O T I N D T I O T C A S I R O I D D
R O U E G R C V O S O O R V N T V O S E I R T R
A A V N M N T E U U V E R S I O N E A R R T I E N
M E D I A C E O M I C L I I T I E T I A O U O
L T N E T V T T N S E T C S H I R V E I E N S I
A E R T E O E S N O S N U O T V T O A L N R I T
T I I I T A T M N D C O V T U E O E O E R N I A
A D E C N C I N R N O E T S S O U R C E A D A D C
G T S S T V E E R T T S H V T D E A A N I C S C I
E V A S C T T N I I T T T O O S T T D G O R A T F
N O L I O N O I T U T I T S N N P T G N E T H T I
E S A E I I G L O E G E L O I D O S R R I I R T
S U T C I D L S I O N A G N N M N C N S V I A N N
T L E N R T S S O T I I T E I T N E E N S R M D R E
V C E I A N I I V A Q E S E N T S S C O D D A D
O E I E E F C E G M R C U N G A E O A R M C U
V A M R R D C O S T I C F O E D N C O T O E E E
O I T O I C L N T S E R S H S E S N I E R N O S R
L A S D R E N D I N E E S S I M A H O C C A I E
O S O V N O I U T C N R O V V V O R S O C N S L E
D T N T U I S I V L S R S S N A I N E O I L G A E
S O A O R N T V S R I T N I E E V N R E A M I G T
A S O H T I G C E N L I G N S N N C G O M O N N R
```

Words List

sponsor	investigator	institution	record
location	essential	source	documents
storage	archiving	media	identification
version	retrieval		

Bonus Trivia Word Search

Solution

Find the answers to these questions in the word search below.

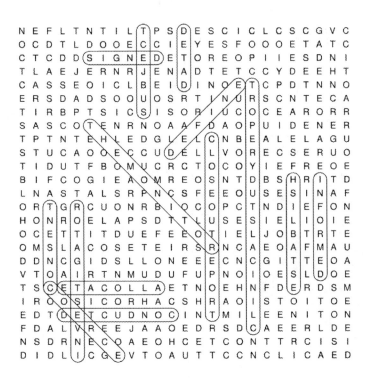

Words List

Allocate	Define	Establish	Investigator
Coerce	Informed	Consent	Dated
Signed	Subject	Conducted	Close out report
Clinical study report	The monitor		

INTERNATIONAL COUNCIL FOR HARMONISATION OF TECHNICAL
REQUIREMENTS FOR PHARMACEUTICALS FOR HUMAN USE (ICH)

ICH HARMONISED GUIDELINE

INTEGRATED ADDENDUM TO ICH E6(R1):
GUIDELINE FOR GOOD CLINICAL PRACTICE

E6(R2)

Current *Step 4* version
dated 9 November 2016

E6(R1)
Document History

First Codification	History	Date	New Codification **November 2005**
E6	Approval by the Steering Committee under *Step 2* and release for public consultation.	27 April 1995	E6
E6	Approval by the Steering Committee under *Step 4* and recommended for adoption to the three ICH regulatory bodies.	1 May 1996	E6

E6(R1) *Step 4* version

E6	Approval by the Steering Committee of *Post-Step 4* editorial corrections.	10 June 1996	E6(R1)

Current E6(R2) Addendum *Step 4* version

Code	History	Date
E6(R2)	Adoption by the Regulatory Members of the ICH Assembly under *Step 4*. Integrated Addendum to ICH E6(R1) document. Changes are integrated directly into the following sections of the parental Guideline: Introduction, 1.63, 1.64, 1.65, 2.10, 2.13, 4.2.5, 4.2.6, 4.9.0, 5.0, 5.0.1, 5.0.2, 5.0.3, 5.0.4, 5.0.5, 5.0.6, 5.0.7, 5.2.2, 5.5.3 (a), 5.5.3 (b), 5.5.3 (h), 5.18.3, 5.18.6 (e), 5.18.7, 5.20.1, 8.1	9 November 2016

or translation of the document, reasonable steps must be taken to clearly label, demarcate or otherwise identify that changes were made to or based on the original document. Any impression that the adaption, modification or translation of the original document is endorsed or sponsored by the ICH must be avoided.

The document is provided "as is" without warranty of any kind. In no event shall the ICH or the authors of the original document be liable for any claim, damages or other liability arising from the use of the document.

The above-mentioned permissions do not apply to content supplied by third parties. Therefore, for documents where the copyright vests in a third party, permission for reproduction must be obtained from this copyright holder.

ICH HARMONISED GUIDELINE

INTEGRATED ADDENDUM TO ICH E6(R1): GUIDELINE FOR GOOD CLINICAL PRACTICE ICH

E6(R2)

ICH Consensus Guideline

INTEGRATED ADDENDUM TO ICH E6(R1): GUIDELINE FOR GOOD CLINICAL PRACTICE ICH

E6(R2)

INTRODUCTION

Good Clinical Practice (GCP) is an international ethical and scientific quality standard for designing, conducting, recording and reporting trials that involve the participation of human subjects. Compliance with this standard provides public assurance that the rights, safety and well-being of trial subjects are protected, consistent with the principles that have their origin in the Declaration of Helsinki, and that the clinical trial data are credible.

The objective of this ICH GCP Guideline is to provide a unified standard for the European Union (EU), Japan and the United States to facilitate the mutual acceptance of clinical data by the regulatory authorities in these jurisdictions.

The guideline was developed with consideration of the current good clinical practices of the European Union, Japan, and the United States, as well as those of Australia, Canada, the Nordic countries and the World Health Organization (WHO).

This guideline should be followed when generating clinical trial data that are intended to be submitted to regulatory authorities.

The principles established in this guideline may also be applied to other clinical investigations that may have an impact on the safety and well-being of human subjects.

ADDENDUM

Since the development of the ICH GCP Guideline, the scale, complexity, and cost of clinical trials have increased. Evolutions in technology and risk management processes offer new opportunities to increase efficiency and focus on relevant activities. When the original ICH E6(R1) text was prepared, clinical trials were performed in a largely paper-based process. Advances in use of electronic data recording and reporting facilitate implementation of other approaches. For example, centralized monitoring can now offer a greater advantage, to a broader range of trials than is suggested in the original text. Therefore, this guideline has been amended to encourage implementation of improved and more efficient approaches to clinical trial design, conduct, oversight, recording and reporting while continuing to ensure human subject protection and reliability of trial results. Standards regarding electronic records and essential documents intended to increase clinical trial quality and efficiency have also been updated.

This guideline should be read in conjunction with other ICH guidelines relevant to the conduct of clinical trials (e.g., E2A (clinical safety data management), E3 (clinical study reporting), E7 (geriatric populations), E8 (general considerations for clinical trials), E9 (statistical principles), and E11 (pediatric populations)).

This ICH GCP Guideline Integrated Addendum provides a unified standard for the European Union, Japan, the United States, Canada, and Switzerland to facilitate the mutual acceptance of data from clinical trials by the regulatory authorities in these jurisdictions. In the event of any conflict between the E6(R1) text and the E6(R2) addendum text, the E6(R2) addendum text should take priority.

1. GLOSSARY

1.1 Adverse Drug Reaction (ADR)

In the pre-approval clinical experience with a new medicinal product or its new usages, particularly as the therapeutic dose(s) may not be established: all noxious and unintended responses to a medicinal product related to any dose should be considered adverse drug reactions. The phrase responses to a medicinal product means that a causal relationship between a medicinal product and an adverse event is at least a reasonable possibility, i.e., the relationship cannot be ruled out.

Regarding marketed medicinal products: a response to a drug which is noxious and unintended and which occurs at doses normally used in man for prophylaxis, diagnosis, or therapy of diseases or for modification of physiological function (see the ICH Guideline for Clinical Safety Data Management: Definitions and Standards for Expedited Reporting).

1.2 Adverse Event (AE)

Any untoward medical occurrence in a patient or clinical investigation subject administered a pharmaceutical product and which does not necessarily have a causal relationship with this treatment. An adverse event (AE) can therefore be any unfavourable and unintended sign (including an abnormal laboratory finding), symptom, or disease temporally associated with the use of a medicinal (investigational) product, whether or not related to the medicinal (investigational) product (see the ICH Guideline for Clinical Safety Data Management: Definitions and Standards for Expedited Reporting).

1.3 Amendment (to the protocol)

See Protocol Amendment.

1.4 Applicable Regulatory Requirement(s)

Any law(s) and regulation(s) addressing the conduct of clinical trials of investigational products.

1.5 Approval (in relation to Institutional Review Boards)

The affirmative decision of the IRB that the clinical trial has been reviewed and may be conducted at the institution site within the constraints set forth by the IRB, the institution, Good Clinical Practice (GCP), and the applicable regulatory requirements.

1.6 Audit

A systematic and independent examination of trial related activities and documents to determine whether the evaluated trial related activities were conducted, and the data were recorded, analyzed and accurately reported according to the protocol, sponsor's standard operating procedures (SOPs), Good Clinical Practice (GCP), and the applicable regulatory requirement(s).

1.7 Audit Certificate

A declaration of confirmation by the auditor that an audit has taken place.

1.8 Audit Report

A written evaluation by the sponsor's auditor of the results of the audit.

1.9 Audit Trail

Documentation that allows reconstruction of the course of events.

1.10 Blinding/Masking

A procedure in which one or more parties to the trial are kept unaware of the treatment assignment(s). Single-blinding usually refers to the subject(s) being unaware, and double- blinding usually refers to the subject(s), investigator(s), monitor, and, in some cases, data analyst(s) being unaware of the treatment assignment(s).

1.11 Case Report Form (CRF)

A printed, optical, or electronic document designed to record all of the protocol required information to be reported to the sponsor on each trial subject.

1.12 Clinical Trial/Study

Any investigation in human subjects intended to discover or verify the clinical, pharmacological and/or other pharmacodynamic effects of an investigational product(s), and/or to identify any adverse reactions to an investigational product(s), and/or to study absorption, distribution, metabolism, and excretion of an investigational product(s) with the object of ascertaining its safety and/or efficacy. The terms clinical trial and clinical study are synonymous.

1.13 Clinical Trial/Study Report

A written description of a trial/study of any therapeutic, prophylactic, or diagnostic agent conducted in human subjects, in which the clinical and statistical description, presentations, and analyses are fully integrated into a single report (see the ICH Guideline for Structure and Content of Clinical Study Reports).

1.14 Comparator (Product)

An investigational or marketed product (i.e., active control), or placebo, used as a reference in a clinical trial.

1.15 Compliance (in relation to trials)

Adherence to all the trial-related requirements, Good Clinical Practice (GCP) requirements, and the applicable regulatory requirements.

1.16 Confidentiality

Prevention of disclosure, to other than authorized individuals, of a sponsor's proprietary information or of a subject's identity.

1.17 Contract

A written, dated, and signed agreement between two or more involved parties that sets out any arrangements on delegation and distribution of tasks and obligations and, if appropriate, on financial matters. The protocol may serve as the basis of a contract.

1.18 Coordinating Committee

A committee that a sponsor may organize to coordinate the conduct of a multicentre trial.

1.19 Coordinating Investigator

An investigator assigned the responsibility for the coordination of investigators at different centres participating in a multicentre trial.

1.20 Contract Research Organization (CRO)

A person or an organization (commercial, academic, or other) contracted by the sponsor to perform one or more of a sponsor's trial-related duties and functions.

1.21 Direct Access

Permission to examine, analyze, verify, and reproduce any records and reports that are important to evaluation of a clinical trial. Any party (e.g., domestic and foreign regulatory authorities, sponsor's monitors and auditors) with direct access should take all reasonable precautions within the constraints of the applicable regulatory requirement(s) to maintain the confidentiality of subjects' identities and sponsor's proprietary information.

1.22 Documentation

All records, in any form (including, but not limited to, written, electronic, magnetic, and optical records, and scans, x-rays, and electrocardiograms) that describe or record the methods, conduct, and/or results of a trial, the factors affecting a trial, and the actions taken.

1.23 Essential Documents

Documents which individually and collectively permit evaluation of the conduct of a study and the quality of the data produced (see 8. Essential Documents for the Conduct of a Clinical Trial).

1.24 Good Clinical Practice (GCP)

A standard for the design, conduct, performance, monitoring, auditing, recording, analyses, and reporting of clinical trials that provides assurance that the data and reported results are credible and accurate, and that the rights, integrity, and confidentiality of trial subjects are protected.

1.25 Independent Data-Monitoring Committee (IDMC) (Data and Safety Monitoring Board, Monitoring Committee, Data Monitoring Committee)

An independent data-monitoring committee that may be established by the sponsor to assess at intervals the progress of a clinical trial, the safety data, and the critical efficacy endpoints, and to recommend to the sponsor whether to continue, modify, or stop a trial.

1.26 Impartial Witness

A person, who is independent of the trial, who cannot be unfairly influenced by people involved with the trial, who attends the informed consent process if the subject or the subject's legally acceptable representative cannot read, and who reads the informed consent form and any other written information supplied to the subject.

1.27 Independent Ethics Committee (IEC)

An independent body (a review board or a committee, institutional, regional, national, or supranational), constituted of medical professionals and non-medical members, whose responsibility it is to ensure the protection of the rights, safety and well-being of human subjects involved in a trial and to provide public assurance of that protection, by, among other things, reviewing and approving/ providing favourable opinion on, the trial protocol, the suitability of the investigator(s), facilities, and the methods and material to be used in obtaining and documenting informed consent of the trial subjects.

The legal status, composition, function, operations and regulatory requirements pertaining to Independent Ethics Committees may differ among countries, but should allow the Independent Ethics Committee to act in agreement with GCP as described in this guideline.

1.28   Informed Consent

A process by which a subject voluntarily confirms his or her willingness to participate in a particular trial, after having been informed of all aspects of the trial that are relevant to the subject's decision to participate. Informed consent is documented by means of a written, signed and dated informed consent form.

1.29   Inspection

The act by a regulatory authority(ies) of conducting an official review of documents, facilities, records, and any other resources that are deemed by the authority(ies) to be related to the clinical trial and that may be located at the site of the trial, at the sponsor's and/or contract research organization's (CRO's) facilities, or at other establishments deemed appropriate by the regulatory authority(ies).

1.30   Institution (medical)

Any public or private entity or agency or medical or dental facility where clinical trials are conducted.

1.31   Institutional Review Board (IRB)

An independent body constituted of medical, scientific, and non-scientific members, whose responsibility is to ensure the protection of the rights, safety and well-being of human subjects involved in a trial by, among other things, reviewing, approving, and providing continuing review of trial protocol and amendments and of the methods and material to be used in obtaining and documenting informed consent of the trial subjects.

1.32   Interim Clinical Trial/Study Report

A report of intermediate results and their evaluation based on analyses performed during the course of a trial.

1.33   Investigational Product

A pharmaceutical form of an active ingredient or placebo being tested or used as a reference in a clinical trial, including a product with a marketing authorization when used or assembled (formulated or packaged) in a way different from the approved form, or when used for an unapproved indication, or when used to gain further information about an approved use.

1.34   Investigator

A person responsible for the conduct of the clinical trial at a trial site. If a trial is conducted by a team of individuals at a trial site, the investigator is the responsible leader of the team and may be called the principal investigator. See also Subinvestigator.

1.35   Investigator/Institution

An expression meaning "the investigator and/or institution, where required by the applicable regulatory requirements".

1.36   Investigator's Brochure

A compilation of the clinical and nonclinical data on the investigational product(s) which is relevant to the study of the investigational product(s) in human subjects (see 7. Investigator's Brochure).

1.37   Legally Acceptable Representative

An individual or juridical or other body authorized under applicable law to consent, on behalf of a prospective subject, to the subject's participation in the clinical trial.

1.38 Monitoring

The act of overseeing the progress of a clinical trial, and of ensuring that it is conducted, recorded, and reported in accordance with the protocol, Standard Operating Procedures (SOPs), Good Clinical Practice (GCP), and the applicable regulatory requirement(s).

1.39 Monitoring Report

A written report from the monitor to the sponsor after each site visit and/or other trial-related communication according to the sponsor's SOPs.

1.40 Multicentre Trial

A clinical trial conducted according to a single protocol but at more than one site, and therefore, carried out by more than one investigator.

1.41 Nonclinical Study

Biomedical studies not performed on human subjects.

1.42 Opinion (in relation to Independent Ethics Committee)

The judgement and/or the advice provided by an Independent Ethics Committee (IEC).

1.43 Original Medical Record

See Source Documents.

1.44 Protocol

A document that describes the objective(s), design, methodology, statistical considerations, and organization of a trial. The protocol usually also gives the background and rationale for the trial, but these could be provided in other protocol referenced documents. Throughout the ICH GCP Guideline the term protocol refers to protocol and protocol amendments.

1.45 Protocol Amendment

A written description of a change(s) to or formal clarification of a protocol.

1.46 Quality Assurance (QA)

All those planned and systematic actions that are established to ensure that the trial is performed and the data are generated, documented (recorded), and reported in compliance with Good Clinical Practice (GCP) and the applicable regulatory requirement(s).

1.47 Quality Control (QC)

The operational techniques and activities undertaken within the quality assurance system to verify that the requirements for quality of the trial-related activities have been fulfilled.

1.48 Randomization

The process of assigning trial subjects to treatment or control groups using an element of chance to determine the assignments in order to reduce bias.

1.49 Regulatory Authorities

Bodies having the power to regulate. In the ICH GCP Guideline the expression Regulatory Authorities includes the authorities that review submitted clinical data and those that conduct inspections (see 1.29). These bodies are sometimes referred to as competent authorities.

1.50 Serious Adverse Event (SAE) or Serious Adverse Drug Reaction (Serious ADR)

Any untoward medical occurrence that at any dose:

- results in death,
- is life-threatening,
- requires inpatient hospitalization or prolongation of existing hospitalization,

- results in persistent or significant disability/incapacity, or
- is a congenital anomaly/birth defect

(see the ICH Guideline for Clinical Safety Data Management: Definitions and Standards for Expedited Reporting).

1.51   Source Data

All information in original records and certified copies of original records of clinical findings, observations, or other activities in a clinical trial necessary for the reconstruction and evaluation of the trial. Source data are contained in source documents (original records or certified copies).

1.52   Source Documents

Original documents, data, and records (e.g., hospital records, clinical and office charts, laboratory notes, memoranda, subjects' diaries or evaluation checklists, pharmacy dispensing records, recorded data from automated instruments, copies or transcriptions certified after verification as being accurate copies, microfiches, photographic negatives, microfilm or magnetic media, x-rays, subject files, and records kept at the pharmacy, at the laboratories and at medico-technical departments involved in the clinical trial).

1.53   Sponsor

An individual, company, institution, or organization which takes responsibility for the initiation, management, and/or financing of a clinical trial.

1.54   Sponsor-Investigator

An individual who both initiates and conducts, alone or with others, a clinical trial, and under whose immediate direction the investigational product is administered to, dispensed to, or used by a subject. The term does not include any person other than an individual (e.g., it does not include a corporation or an agency). The obligations of a sponsor-investigator include both those of a sponsor and those of an investigator.

1.55 Standard Operating Procedures (SOPs)

Detailed, written instructions to achieve uniformity of the performance of a specific function.

1.56 Subinvestigator

Any individual member of the clinical trial team designated and supervised by the investigator at a trial site to perform critical trial-related procedures and/or to make important trial-related decisions (e.g., associates, residents, research fellows). See also Investigator.

1.57 Subject/Trial Subject

An individual who participates in a clinical trial, either as a recipient of the investigational product(s) or as a control.

1.58 Subject Identification Code

A unique identifier assigned by the investigator to each trial subject to protect the subject's identity and used in lieu of the subject's name when the investigator reports adverse events and/or other trial related data.

1.59 Trial Site

The location(s) where trial-related activities are actually conducted.

1.60 Unexpected Adverse Drug Reaction

An adverse reaction, the nature or severity of which is not consistent with the applicable product information (e.g., Investigator's Brochure for an unapproved investigational product or package insert/summary of product characteristics for an approved product) (see the ICH Guideline for Clinical Safety Data Management: Definitions and Standards for Expedited Reporting).

1.61 Vulnerable Subjects

Individuals whose willingness to volunteer in a clinical trial may be unduly influenced by the expectation, whether justified or not, of benefits associated with participation, or of a retaliatory response from senior members of a hierarchy in case of refusal to participate. Examples are members of a group with a hierarchical structure, such as medical, pharmacy, dental, and nursing students, subordinate hospital and laboratory personnel, employees of the pharmaceutical industry, members of the armed forces, and persons kept in detention. Other vulnerable subjects include patients with incurable diseases, persons in nursing homes, unemployed or impoverished persons, patients in emergency situations, ethnic minority groups, homeless persons, nomads, refugees, minors, and those incapable of giving consent.

1.62   Well-being (of the trial subjects)

The physical and mental integrity of the subjects participating in a clinical trial.

ADDENDUM

1.63   Certified Copy

A copy (irrespective of the type of media used) of the original record that has been verified (i.e., by a dated signature or by generation through a validated process) to have the same information, including data that describe the context, content, and structure, as the original.

1.64   Monitoring Plan

A document that describes the strategy, methods, responsibilities, and requirements for monitoring the trial.

1.65   Validation of Computerized Systems

A process of establishing and documenting that the specified requirements of a computerized system can be consistently fulfilled from design until decommissioning of the system or transition to a new system. The approach to validation should be based on a risk assessment that takes into consideration the intended use of the system and the potential of the system to affect human subject protection and reliability of trial results.

2. THE PRINCIPLES OF ICH GCP

2.1 Clinical trials should be conducted in accordance with the ethical principles that have their origin in the Declaration of Helsinki, and that are consistent with GCP and the applicable regulatory requirement(s).

2.2 Before a trial is initiated, foreseeable risks and inconveniences should be weighed against the anticipated benefit for the individual trial subject and society. A trial should be initiated and continued only if the anticipated benefits justify the risks.

2.3 The rights, safety, and well-being of the trial subjects are the most important considerations and should prevail over interests of science and society.

2.4 The available nonclinical and clinical information on an investigational product should be adequate to support the proposed clinical trial.

2.5 Clinical trials should be scientifically sound, and described in a clear, detailed protocol.

2.6 A trial should be conducted in compliance with the protocol that has received prior institutional review board (IRB)/ independent ethics committee (IEC) approval/favorable opinion.

2.7 The medical care given to, and medical decisions made on behalf of, subjects should always be the responsibility of a qualified physician or, when appropriate, of a qualified dentist.

2.8 Each individual involved in conducting a trial should be qualified by education, training, and experience to perform his or her respective task(s).

2.9 Freely given informed consent should be obtained from every subject prior to clinical trial participation.

2.10 All clinical trial information should be recorded, handled, and stored in a way that allows its accurate reporting, interpretation and verification.

ADDENDUM

This principle applies to all records referenced in this guideline, irrespective of the type of media used.

2.11 The confidentiality of records that could identify subjects should be protected, respecting the privacy and confidentiality rules in accordance with the applicable regulatory requirement(s).

2.12 Investigational products should be manufactured, handled, and stored in accordance with applicable good manufacturing practice (GMP). They should be used in accordance with the approved protocol.

2.13 Systems with procedures that assure the quality of every aspect of the trial should be implemented.

ADDENDUM

Aspects of the trial that are essential to ensure human subject protection and reliability of trial results should be the focus of such systems.

3. INSTITUTIONAL REVIEW BOARD/ INDEPENDENT ETHICS COMMITTEE (IRB/IEC)

3.1 Responsibilities

3.1.1 An IRB/IEC should safeguard the rights, safety, and well-being of all trial subjects. Special attention should be paid to trials that may include vulnerable subjects.

3.1.2 The IRB/IEC should obtain the following documents:

trial protocol(s)/amendment(s), written informed consent form(s) and consent form updates that the investigator proposes for use in the trial, subject recruitment procedures (e.g., advertisements), written information to be provided to subjects, Investigator's Brochure (IB), available safety information, information about payments and compensation available to subjects, the investigator's current curriculum vitae and/or other documentation evidencing qualifications, and any other documents that the IRB/IEC may need to fulfil its responsibilities.

The IRB/IEC should review a proposed clinical trial within a reasonable time and document its views in writing, clearly identifying the trial, the documents reviewed and the dates for the following:

- approval/favorable opinion;
- modifications required prior to its approval/favorable opinion;
- disapproval / negative opinion; and
- termination/suspension of any prior approval/favorable opinion.

3.1.3   The IRB/IEC should consider the qualifications of the investigator for the proposed trial, as documented by a current curriculum vitae and/or by any other relevant documentation the IRB/IEC requests.

3.1.4   The IRB/IEC should conduct continuing review of each ongoing trial at intervals appropriate to the degree of risk to human subjects, but at least once per year.

3.1.5   The IRB/IEC may request more information than is outlined in paragraph 4.8.10 be given to subjects when, in the judgement of the IRB/IEC, the additional information would add meaningfully to the protection of the rights, safety and/or well-being of the subjects.

3.1.6   When a non-therapeutic trial is to be carried out with the consent of the subject's legally acceptable representative (see 4.8.12, 4.8.14), the IRB/IEC should determine that the proposed protocol and/or other document(s) adequately addresses relevant ethical concerns and meets applicable regulatory requirements for such trials.

3.1.7   Where the protocol indicates that prior consent of the trial subject or the subject's legally acceptable representative is not possible (see 4.8.15), the IRB/IEC should determine that the proposed protocol and/or other document(s) adequately addresses relevant ethical concerns and meets applicable regulatory requirements for such trials (i.e., in emergency situations).

3.1.8   The IRB/IEC should review both the amount and method of payment to subjects to assure that neither presents problems of coercion or undue influence on the trial subjects. Payments to a subject should be prorated and not wholly contingent on completion of the trial by the subject.

3.1.9   The IRB/IEC should ensure that information regarding payment to subjects, including the methods, amounts, and schedule of payment to trial subjects, is set forth in the written informed consent form and any other written information to be provided to subjects. The way payment will be prorated should be specified.

3.2   Composition, Functions and Operations

3.2.1   The IRB/IEC should consist of a reasonable number of members, who collectively have the qualifications and experience to review and evaluate the science, medical

aspects, and ethics of the proposed trial. It is recommended that the IRB/IEC should include:

(a) At least five members.
(b) At least one member whose primary area of interest is in a nonscientific area.
(c) At least one member who is independent of the institution/ trial site.

Only those IRB/IEC members who are independent of the investigator and the sponsor of the trial should vote/provide opinion on a trial-related matter.

A list of IRB/IEC members and their qualifications should be maintained.

3.2.2   The IRB/IEC should perform its functions according to written operating procedures, should maintain written records of its activities and minutes of its meetings, and should comply with GCP and with the applicable regulatory requirement(s).

3.2.3   An IRB/IEC should make its decisions at announced meetings at which at least a quorum, as stipulated in its written operating procedures, is present.

3.2.4   Only members who participate in the IRB/IEC review and discussion should vote/provide their opinion and/or advise.

3.2.5   The investigator may provide information on any aspect of the trial, but should not participate in the deliberations of the IRB/IEC or in the vote/opinion of the IRB/IEC.

3.2.6   An IRB/IEC may invite nonmembers with expertise in special areas for assistance.

3.3 Procedures

The IRB/IEC should establish, document in writing, and follow its procedures, which should include:

3.3.1   Determining its composition (names and qualifications of the members) and the authority under which it is established.

3.3.2   Scheduling, notifying its members of, and conducting its meetings.

3.3.3   Conducting initial and continuing review of trials.

3.3.4   Determining the frequency of continuing review, as appropriate.

3.3.5   Providing, according to the applicable regulatory requirements, expedited review and approval/favorable opinion of minor change(s) in ongoing trials that have the approval/favorable opinion of the IRB/IEC.

3.3.6   Specifying that no subject should be admitted to a trial before the IRB/IEC issues its written approval/favorable opinion of the trial.

3.3.7   Specifying that no deviations from, or changes of, the protocol should be initiated without prior written IRB/IEC approval/ favorable opinion of an appropriate amendment, except when necessary to eliminate immediate hazards to the subjects or when the change(s) involves only logistical or administrative aspects of the trial (e.g., change of monitor(s), telephone number(s)) (see 4.5.2).

3.3.8   Specifying that the investigator should promptly report to the IRB/IEC:

(a)   Deviations from, or changes of, the protocol to eliminate immediate hazards to the trial subjects (see 3.3.7, 4.5.2, 4.5.4).

(b)   Changes increasing the risk to subjects and/or affecting significantly the conduct of the trial (see 4.10.2).

(c)   All adverse drug reactions (ADRs) that are both serious and unexpected.

(d)   New information that may affect adversely the safety of the subjects or the conduct of the trial.

3.3.9   Ensuring that the IRB/IEC promptly notify in writing the investigator/institution concerning:

(a)   Its trial-related decisions/opinions.

(b)   The reasons for its decisions/opinions.

(c)   Procedures for appeal of its decisions/opinions.

3.4   Records

The IRB/IEC should retain all relevant records (e.g., written procedures, membership lists, lists of occupations/affiliations of members, submitted documents, minutes of meetings, and correspondence) for a period of at least 3-years after completion of the trial and make them available upon request from the regulatory authority(ies).

The IRB/IEC may be asked by investigators, sponsors or regulatory authorities to provide its written procedures and membership lists.

4. INVESTIGATOR

4.1 Investigator's Qualifications and Agreements

4.1.1   The investigator(s) should be qualified by education, training, and experience to assume responsibility for the proper conduct of the trial, should meet all the qualifications specified by the applicable regulatory requirement(s), and should provide evidence of such qualifications through up-to-date curriculum vitae and/or other relevant documentation requested by the sponsor, the IRB/IEC, and/or the regulatory authority(ies).

4.1.2   The investigator should be thoroughly familiar with the appropriate use of the investigational product(s), as described in the protocol, in the current Investigator's Brochure, in the product information and in other information sources provided by the sponsor.

4.1.3   The investigator should be aware of, and should comply with, GCP and the applicable regulatory requirements.

4.1.4   The investigator/institution should permit monitoring and auditing by the sponsor, and inspection by the appropriate regulatory authority(ies).

4.1.5   The investigator should maintain a list of appropriately qualified persons to whom the investigator has delegated significant trial-related duties.

4.2 Adequate Resources

4.2.1   The investigator should be able to demonstrate (e.g., based on retrospective data) a potential for recruiting the required number of suitable subjects within the agreed recruitment period.

4.2.2   The investigator should have sufficient time to properly conduct and complete the trial within the agreed trial period.

4.2.3   The investigator should have available an adequate number of qualified staff and adequate facilities for the foreseen duration of the trial to conduct the trial properly and safely.

4.2.4   The investigator should ensure that all persons assisting with the trial are adequately informed about the protocol, the investigational product(s), and their trial-related duties and functions.

ADDENDUM

4.2.5   The investigator is responsible for supervising any individual or party to whom the investigator delegates trial-related duties and functions conducted at the trial site.

4.2.6   If the investigator/institution retains the services of any individual or party to perform trial-related duties and functions, the investigator/institution should ensure this individual or party is qualified to perform those trial-related duties and functions and should implement procedures to ensure the integrity of the trial-related duties and functions performed and any data generated.

4.3   Medical Care of Trial Subjects

4.3.1   A qualified physician (or dentist, when appropriate), who is an investigator or a sub- investigator for the trial, should be responsible for all trial-related medical (or dental) decisions.

4.3.2   During and following a subject's participation in a trial, the investigator/institution should ensure that adequate medical care is provided to a subject for any adverse events, including clinically significant laboratory values, related to the trial. The investigator/institution should inform a subject when medical care is needed for intercurrent illness(es) of which the investigator becomes aware.

4.3.3   It is recommended that the investigator inform the subject's primary physician about the subject's participation in the trial if the subject has a primary physician and if the subject agrees to the primary physician being informed.

4.3.4   Although a subject is not obliged to give his/her reason(s) for withdrawing prematurely from a trial, the investigator should make a reasonable effort to ascertain the reason(s), while fully respecting the subject's rights.

4.4   Communication with IRB/IEC

4.4.1   Before initiating a trial, the investigator/institution should have written and dated approval/favorable opinion from the IRB/IEC for the trial protocol, written informed consent form, consent form updates, subject recruitment procedures (e.g., advertisements), and any other written information to be provided to subjects.

4.4.2   As part of the investigator's/institution's written application to the IRB/IEC, the investigator/institution should provide the IRB/IEC with a current copy of the Investigator's Brochure. If the Investigator's Brochure is updated during the trial, the investigator/institution should supply a copy of the updated Investigator's Brochure to the IRB/IEC.

4.4.3   During the trial the investigator/institution should provide to the IRB/IEC all documents subject to review.

4.5   Compliance with Protocol

4.5.1   The investigator/institution should conduct the trial in compliance with the protocol agreed to by the sponsor and, if required, by the regulatory authority(ies) and which was given approval/favorable opinion by the IRB/IEC. The investigator/institution and the sponsor should sign the protocol, or an alternative contract, to confirm agreement.

4.5.2   The investigator should not implement any deviation from, or changes of the protocol without agreement by the sponsor and prior review and documented approval/favorable opinion from the IRB/IEC of an amendment, except where necessary to eliminate an immediate hazard(s) to trial subjects, or when the change(s) involves only logistical or administrative aspects of the trial (e.g., change in monitor(s), change of telephone number(s)).

4.5.3   The investigator, or person designated by the investigator, should document and explain any deviation from the approved protocol.

4.5.4   The investigator may implement a deviation from, or a change of, the protocol to eliminate an immediate hazard(s) to trial subjects without prior IRB/IEC approval/favorable opinion. As soon as possible, the implemented deviation or change, the reasons for it, and, if appropriate, the proposed protocol amendment(s) should be submitted:

(a)   to the IRB/IEC for review and approval/favorable opinion,
(b)   to the sponsor for agreement and, if required,
(c)   to the regulatory authority(ies).

4.6   Investigational Product(s)

4.6.1   Responsibility for investigational product(s) accountability at the trial site(s) rests with the investigator/institution.

4.6.2   Where allowed/required, the investigator/institution may/ should assign some or all of the investigator's/institution's duties for investigational product(s) accountability at the trial site(s) to an appropriate pharmacist or another appropriate individual who is under the supervision of the investigator/ institution.

4.6.3   The investigator/institution and/or a pharmacist or other appropriate individual, who is designated by the investigator/ institution, should maintain records of the product's delivery to the trial site, the inventory at the site, the use by each subject, and the return to the sponsor or alternative disposition of unused product(s). These records should include dates, quantities, batch/serial numbers, expiration dates (if applicable), and the unique code numbers assigned to the investigational product(s) and trial subjects. Investigators should maintain records that document adequately that the subjects were provided the doses specified by the protocol and reconcile all investigational product(s) received from the sponsor.

4.6.4   The investigational product(s) should be stored as specified by the sponsor (see 5.13.2 and 5.14.3) and in accordance with applicable regulatory requirement(s).

4.6.5   The investigator should ensure that the investigational product(s) are used only in accordance with the approved protocol.

4.6.6   The investigator, or a person designated by the investigator/ institution, should explain the correct use of the investigational product(s) to each subject and should check, at intervals appropriate for the trial, that each subject is following the instructions properly.

4.7   Randomization Procedures and Unblinding

The investigator should follow the trial's randomization procedures, if any, and should ensure that the code is broken only in accordance with the protocol. If the trial is blinded, the investigator should promptly document and explain to the sponsor any premature unblinding (e.g., accidental unblinding, unblinding due to a serious adverse event) of the investigational product(s).

4.8   Informed Consent of Trial Subjects

4.8.1   In obtaining and documenting informed consent, the investigator should comply with the applicable regulatory requirement(s), and should adhere to GCP and to the ethical principles that have their origin in the Declaration of Helsinki. Prior to the beginning of the trial, the investigator should have the IRB/IEC's written approval/favorable opinion of the written informed consent form and any other written information to be provided to subjects.

4.8.2   The written informed consent form and any other written information to be provided to subjects should be revised whenever important new information becomes available that may be relevant to the subject's consent. Any revised written informed consent form, and written information should receive the IRB/IEC's approval/favorable opinion in advance of use. The subject or the subject's legally acceptable representative should be informed in a timely manner if new information becomes available that may be relevant to the subject's willingness to continue participation in the trial. The communication of this information should be documented.

4.8.3   Neither the investigator, nor the trial staff, should coerce or unduly influence a subject to participate or to continue to participate in a trial.

4.8.4   None of the oral and written information concerning the trial, including the written informed consent form, should contain any language that causes the subject or the subject's legally acceptable representative to waive or to appear to waive any legal rights, or that releases or appears to release the investigator, the institution, the sponsor, or their agents from liability for negligence.

4.8.5   The investigator, or a person designated by the investigator, should fully inform the subject or, if the subject is unable to provide informed consent, the subject's legally acceptable representative, of all pertinent aspects of the trial including the written information and the approval/ favorable opinion by the IRB/IEC.

4.8.6   The language used in the oral and written information about the trial, including the written informed consent form, should be as non-technical as practical and should be understandable to the subject or the subject's legally acceptable representative and the impartial witness, where applicable.

4.8.7   Before informed consent may be obtained, the investigator, or a person designated by the investigator, should provide the subject or the subject's legally acceptable representative ample time and opportunity to inquire about details of the trial and to decide whether or not to participate in the trial. All questions about the trial should be answered to the satisfaction of the subject or the subject's legally acceptable representative.

4.8.8   Prior to a subject's participation in the trial, the written informed consent form should be signed and personally dated by the subject or by the subject's legally acceptable representative, and by the person who conducted the informed consent discussion.

4.8.9   If a subject is unable to read or if a legally acceptable representative is unable to read, an impartial witness should be present during the entire informed consent discussion. After the written informed consent form and any other written information to be provided to subjects, is read and explained to the subject or the subject's legally acceptable representative, and after the subject or the subject's legally acceptable representative has orally consented to the subject's participation in the trial and, if capable of doing so, has signed and personally dated the informed consent form, the witness should sign and personally date the consent form. By signing the consent form, the witness attests that the information in the consent form and any other written information was accurately explained to, and apparently understood by, the subject or the subject's legally acceptable representative, and that informed consent was freely given by the subject or the subject's legally acceptable representative.

4.8.10   Both the informed consent discussion and the written informed consent form and any other written information to be provided to subjects should include explanations of the following:

(a)   That the trial involves research.

(b)   The purpose of the trial.

(c)   The trial treatment(s) and the probability for random assignment to each treatment.

(d)   The trial procedures to be followed, including all invasive procedures.

(e)   The subject's responsibilities.

(f)   Those aspects of the trial that are experimental.

(g)   The reasonably foreseeable risks or inconveniences to the subject and, when applicable, to an embryo, fetus, or nursing infant.

(h) The reasonably expected benefits. When there is no intended clinical benefit to the subject, the subject should be made aware of this.

(i) The alternative procedure(s) or course(s) of treatment that may be available to the subject, and their important potential benefits and risks.

(j) The compensation and/or treatment available to the subject in the event of trial- related injury.

(k) The anticipated prorated payment, if any, to the subject for participating in the trial.

(l) The anticipated expenses, if any, to the subject for participating in the trial.

(m) That the subject's participation in the trial is voluntary and that the subject may refuse to participate or withdraw from the trial, at any time, without penalty or loss of benefits to which the subject is otherwise entitled.

(n) That the monitor(s), the auditor(s), the IRB/IEC, and the regulatory authority(ies) will be granted direct access to the subject's original medical records for verification of clinical trial procedures and/or data, without violating the confidentiality of the subject, to the extent permitted by the applicable laws and regulations and that, by signing a written informed consent form, the subject or the subject's legally acceptable representative is authorizing such access.

(o) That records identifying the subject will be kept confidential and, to the extent permitted by the applicable laws and/or regulations, will not be made publicly available. If the results of the trial are published, the subject's identity will remain confidential.

(p) That the subject or the subject's legally acceptable representative will be informed in a timely manner if information becomes available that may be relevant to the subject's willingness to continue participation in the trial.

(q) The person(s) to contact for further information regarding the trial and the rights of trial subjects, and whom to contact in the event of trial-related injury.

(r)   The foreseeable circumstances and/or reasons under which the subject's participation in the trial may be terminated.

(s)   The expected duration of the subject's participation in the trial.

(t)   The approximate number of subjects involved in the trial.

4.8.11   Prior to participation in the trial, the subject or the subject's legally acceptable representative should receive a copy of the signed and dated written informed consent form and any other written information provided to the subjects. During a subject's participation in the trial, the subject or the subject's legally acceptable representative should receive a copy of the signed and dated consent form updates and a copy of any amendments to the written information provided to subjects.

4.8.12   When a clinical trial (therapeutic or non-therapeutic) includes subjects who can only be enrolled in the trial with the consent of the subject's legally acceptable representative (e.g., minors, or patients with severe dementia), the subject should be informed about the trial to the extent compatible with the subject's understanding and, if capable, the subject should sign and personally date the written informed consent.

4.8.13   Except as described in 4.8.14, a non-therapeutic trial (i.e., a trial in which there is no anticipated direct clinical benefit to the subject), should be conducted in subjects who personally give consent and who sign and date the written informed consent form.

4.8.14   Non-therapeutic trials may be conducted in subjects with consent of a legally acceptable representative provided the following conditions are fulfilled:

(a)   The objectives of the trial can not be met by means of a trial in subjects who can give informed consent personally.

(b)   The foreseeable risks to the subjects are low.

(c)   The negative impact on the subject's well-being is minimized and low.

(d) The trial is not prohibited by law.

(e) The approval/favorable opinion of the IRB/IEC is expressly sought on the inclusion of such subjects, and the written approval/ favorable opinion covers this aspect.

Such trials, unless an exception is justified, should be conducted in patients having a disease or condition for which the investigational product is intended. Subjects in these trials should be particularly closely monitored and should be withdrawn if they appear to be unduly distressed.

4.8.15   In emergency situations, when prior consent of the subject is not possible, the consent of the subject's legally acceptable representative, if present, should be requested. When prior consent of the subject is not possible, and the subject's legally acceptable representative is not available, enrolment of the subject should require measures described in the protocol and/or elsewhere, with documented approval/favorable opinion by the IRB/IEC, to protect the rights, safety and well-being of the subject and to ensure compliance with applicable regulatory requirements. The subject or the subject's legally acceptable representative should be informed about the trial as soon as possible and consent to continue and other consent as appropriate (see 4.8.10) should be requested.

4.9   Records and Reports

ADDENDUM

4.9.0   The investigator/institution should maintain adequate and accurate source documents and trial records that include all pertinent observations on each of the site's trial subjects. Source data should be attributable, legible, contemporaneous, original, accurate, and complete. Changes to source data should be traceable, should not obscure the original entry, and should be explained if necessary (e.g., *via* an audit trail).

4.9.1   The investigator should ensure the accuracy, completeness, legibility, and timeliness of the data reported to the sponsor in the CRFs and in all required reports.

4.9.2   Data reported on the CRF, that are derived from source documents, should be consistent with the source documents or the discrepancies should be explained.

4.9.3   Any change or correction to a CRF should be dated, initialed, and explained (if necessary) and should not obscure the original entry (i.e., an audit trail should be maintained); this applies to both written and electronic changes or corrections (see 5.18.4 (n)). Sponsors should provide guidance to investigators and/ or the investigators' designated representatives on making such corrections. Sponsors should have written procedures to assure that changes or corrections in CRFs made by sponsor's designated representatives are documented, are necessary, and are endorsed by the investigator. The investigator should retain records of the changes and corrections.

4.9.4   The investigator/institution should maintain the trial documents as specified in Essential Documents for the Conduct of a Clinical Trial (see 8.) and as required by the applicable regulatory requirement(s). The investigator/ institution should take measures to prevent accidental or premature destruction of these documents.

4.9.5   Essential documents should be retained until at least 2-years after the last approval of a marketing application in an ICH region and until there are no pending or contemplated marketing applications in an ICH region or at least 2-years have elapsed since the formal discontinuation of clinical development of the investigational product. These documents should be retained for a longer period however if required by the applicable regulatory requirements or by an agreement with the sponsor. It is the responsibility of the sponsor to inform the investigator/institution as to when these documents no longer need to be retained (see 5.5.12).

4.9.6   The financial aspects of the trial should be documented in an agreement between the sponsor and the investigator/ institution.

4.9.7   Upon request of the monitor, auditor, IRB/IEC, or regulatory authority, the investigator/institution should make available for direct access all requested trial-related records.

4.10   Progress Reports

4.10.1   The investigator should submit written summaries of the trial status to the IRB/IEC annually, or more frequently, if requested by the IRB/IEC.

4.10.2   The investigator should promptly provide written reports to the sponsor, the IRB/IEC (see 3.3.8) and, where applicable, the institution on any changes significantly affecting the conduct of the trial, and/or increasing the risk to subjects.

4.11   Safety Reporting

4.11.1   All serious adverse events (SAEs) should be reported immediately to the sponsor except for those SAEs that the protocol or other document (e.g., Investigator's Brochure) identifies as not needing immediate reporting. The immediate reports should be followed promptly by detailed, written reports. The immediate and follow-up reports should identify subjects by unique code numbers assigned to the trial subjects rather than by the subjects' names, personal identification numbers, and/or addresses. The investigator should also comply with the applicable regulatory requirement(s) related to the reporting of unexpected serious adverse drug reactions to the regulatory authority(ies) and the IRB/IEC.

4.11.2   Adverse events and/or laboratory abnormalities identified in the protocol as critical to safety evaluations should be reported to the sponsor according to the reporting requirements and within the time periods specified by the sponsor in the protocol.

4.11.3   For reported deaths, the investigator should supply the sponsor and the IRB/IEC with any additional requested information (e.g., autopsy reports and terminal medical reports).

4.12 Premature Termination or Suspension of a Trial

If the trial is prematurely terminated or suspended for any reason, the investigator/institution should promptly inform the trial subjects, should assure appropriate therapy and follow-up for the subjects, and, where required by the applicable regulatory requirement(s), should inform the regulatory authority(ies). In addition:

4.12.1   If the investigator terminates or suspends a trial without prior agreement of the sponsor, the investigator should inform the institution where applicable, and the investigator/institution should promptly inform the sponsor and the IRB/IEC, and should provide the sponsor and the IRB/IEC a detailed written explanation of the termination or suspension.

4.12.2   If the sponsor terminates or suspends a trial (see 5.21), the investigator should promptly inform the institution where applicable and the investigator/institution should promptly inform the IRB/IEC and provide the IRB/IEC a detailed written explanation of the termination or suspension.

4.12.3   If the IRB/IEC terminates or suspends its approval/favorable opinion of a trial (see 3.1.2 and 3.3.9), the investigator should inform the institution where applicable and the investigator/ institution should promptly notify the sponsor and provide the sponsor with a detailed written explanation of the termination or suspension.

4.13 Final Report(s) by Investigator

Upon completion of the trial, the investigator, where applicable, should inform the institution; the investigator/institution should provide the IRB/IEC with a summary of the trial's outcome, and the regulatory authority(ies) with any reports required.

5. SPONSOR

ADDENDUM

5.0   Quality Management

The sponsor should implement a system to manage quality throughout all stages of the trial process.

Sponsors should focus on trial activities essential to ensuring human subject protection and the reliability of trial results. Quality management includes the design of efficient clinical trial protocols and tools and procedures for data collection and processing, as well as the collection of information that is essential to decision making.

The methods used to assure and control the quality of the trial should be proportionate to the risks inherent in the trial and the importance of the information collected. The sponsor should ensure that all aspects of the trial are operationally feasible and should avoid unnecessary complexity, procedures, and data collection. Protocols, case report forms, and other operational documents should be clear, concise, and consistent.

The quality management system should use a risk-based approach as described below.

5.0.1   *Critical Process and Data Identification*

During protocol development, the sponsor should identify those processes and data that are critical to ensure human subject protection and the reliability of trial results.

5.0.2   *Risk Identification*

The sponsor should identify risks to critical trial processes and data. Risks should be considered at both the system level (e.g., standard operating procedures, computerized systems, personnel) and clinical trial level (e.g., trial design, data collection, informed consent process).

5.0.3 Risk Evaluation

The sponsor should evaluate the identified risks, against existing risk controls by considering:

(a) The likelihood of errors occurring.

(b) The extent to which such errors would be detectable.

(c) The impact of such errors on human subject protection and reliability of trial results.

5.0.4 Risk Control

The sponsor should decide which risks to reduce and/or which risks to accept. The approach used to reduce risk to an acceptable level should be proportionate to the significance of the risk. Risk reduction activities may be incorporated in protocol design and implementation, monitoring plans, agreements between parties defining roles and responsibilities, systematic safeguards to ensure adherence to standard operating procedures, and training in processes and procedures.

Predefined quality tolerance limits should be established, taking into consideration the medical and statistical characteristics of the variables as well as the statistical design of the trial, to identify systematic issues that can impact subject safety or reliability of trial results. Detection of deviations from the predefined quality tolerance limits should trigger an evaluation to determine if action is needed.

5.0.5 Risk Communication

The sponsor should document quality management activities. The sponsor should communicate quality management activities to those who are involved in or affected by such activities, to facilitate risk review and continual improvement during clinical trial execution.

5.0.6 Risk Review

The sponsor should periodically review risk control measures to ascertain whether the implemented quality management activities remain effective and relevant, taking into account emerging knowledge and experience.

5.0.7   Risk Reporting

The sponsor should describe the quality management approach implemented in the trial and summarize important deviations from the predefined quality tolerance limits and remedial actions taken in the clinical study report (ICH E3, Section 9.6 Data Quality Assurance).

5.1   Quality Assurance and Quality Control

5.1.1   The sponsor is responsible for implementing and maintaining quality assurance and quality control systems with written SOPs to ensure that trials are conducted and data are generated, documented (recorded), and reported in compliance with the protocol, GCP, and the applicable regulatory requirement(s).

5.1.2   The sponsor is responsible for securing agreement from all involved parties to ensure direct access (see 1.21) to all trial related sites, source data/documents, and reports for the purpose of monitoring and auditing by the sponsor, and inspection by domestic and foreign regulatory authorities.

5.1.3   Quality control should be applied to each stage of data handling to ensure that all data are reliable and have been processed correctly.

5.1.4   Agreements, made by the sponsor with the investigator/ institution and any other parties involved with the clinical trial, should be in writing, as part of the protocol or in a separate agreement.

5.2   Contract Research Organization (CRO)

5.2.1   A sponsor may transfer any or all of the sponsor's trial-related duties and functions to a CRO, but the ultimate responsibility for the quality and integrity of the trial data always resides with the sponsor. The CRO should implement quality assurance and quality control.

5.2.2   Any trial-related duty and function that is transferred to and assumed by a CRO should be specified in writing.

ADDENDUM

The sponsor should ensure oversight of any trial-related duties and functions carried out on its behalf, including trial-related duties and functions that are subcontracted to another party by the sponsor's contracted CRO(s).

5.2.3   Any trial-related duties and functions not specifically transferred to and assumed by a CRO are retained by the sponsor.

5.2.4   All references to a sponsor in this guideline also apply to a CRO to the extent that a CRO has assumed the trial related duties and functions of a sponsor.

5.3   Medical Expertise

The sponsor should designate appropriately qualified medical personnel who will be readily available to advise on trial related medical questions or problems. If necessary, outside consultant(s) may be appointed for this purpose.

5.4   Trial Design

5.4.1   The sponsor should utilize qualified individuals (e.g., biostatisticians, clinical pharmacologists, and physicians) as appropriate, throughout all stages of the trial process, from designing the protocol and CRFs and planning the analyses to analyzing and preparing interim and final clinical trial reports.

5.4.2   For further guidance: Clinical Trial Protocol and Protocol Amendment(s) (see 6.), the ICH Guideline for Structure and Content of Clinical Study Reports, and other appropriate ICH guidance on trial design, protocol and conduct.

5.5   Trial Management, Data Handling, and Record Keeping

5.5.1   The sponsor should utilize appropriately qualified individuals to supervise the overall conduct of the trial, to handle the data, to verify the data, to conduct the statistical analyses, and to prepare the trial reports.

5.5.2   The sponsor may consider establishing an independent data-monitoring committee (IDMC) to assess the progress of a clinical trial, including the safety data and the critical efficacy endpoints at intervals, and to recommend to the sponsor whether to continue, modify, or stop a trial. The IDMC should have written operating procedures and maintain written records of all its meetings.

5.5.3   When using electronic trial data handling and/or remote electronic trial data systems, the sponsor should:

(a)   Ensure and document that the electronic data processing system(s) conforms to the sponsor's established requirements for completeness, accuracy, reliability, and consistent intended performance (i.e., validation).

ADDENDUM

The sponsor should base their approach to validation of such systems on a risk assessment that takes into consideration the intended use of the system and the potential of the system to affect human subject protection and reliability of trial results.

(b)   Maintains SOPs for using these systems.

ADDENDUM

The SOPs should cover system setup, installation, and use. The SOPs should describe system validation and functionality testing, data collection and handling, system maintenance, system security measures, change control, data backup, recovery, contingency planning, and decommissioning. The responsibilities of the sponsor, investigator, and other parties with respect to the use of these computerized systems should be clear, and the users should be provided with training in their use.

(c) Ensure that the systems are designed to permit data changes in such a way that the data changes are documented and that there is no deletion of entered data (i.e., maintain an audit trail, data trail, edit trail).

(d) Maintain a security system that prevents unauthorized access to the data.

(e) Maintain a list of the individuals who are authorized to make data changes (see 4.1.5 and 4.9.3).

(f) Maintain adequate backup of the data.

(g) Safeguard the blinding, if any (e.g., maintain the blinding during data entry and processing).

ADDENDUM

(h) Ensure the integrity of the data including any data that describe the context, content, and structure. This is particularly important when making changes to the computerized systems, such as software upgrades or migration of data.

5.5.4   If data are transformed during processing, it should always be possible to compare the original data and observations with the processed data.

5.5.5   The sponsor should use an unambiguous subject identification code (see 1.58) that allows identification of all the data reported for each subject.

5.5.6   The sponsor, or other owners of the data, should retain all of the sponsor-specific essential documents pertaining to the trial (see 8. Essential Documents for the Conduct of a Clinical Trial).

5.5.7   The sponsor should retain all sponsor-specific essential documents in conformance with the applicable regulatory requirement(s) of the country(ies) where the product is approved, and/or where the sponsor intends to apply for approval(s).

5.5.8   If the sponsor discontinues the clinical development of an investigational product (i.e., for any or all indications, routes of administration, or dosage forms), the sponsor should maintain all sponsor-specific essential documents for at least 2-years after formal discontinuation or in conformance with the applicable regulatory requirement(s).

5.5.9   If the sponsor discontinues the clinical development of an investigational product, the sponsor should notify all the trial investigators/institutions and all the regulatory authorities.

5.5.10   Any transfer of ownership of the data should be reported to the appropriate authority(ies), as required by the applicable regulatory requirement(s).

5.5.11   The sponsor specific essential documents should be retained until at least 2-years after the last approval of a marketing application in an ICH region and until there are no pending or contemplated marketing applications in an ICH region or at least 2-years have elapsed since the formal discontinuation of clinical development of the investigational product. These documents should be retained for a longer period however if required by the applicable regulatory requirement(s) or if needed by the sponsor.

5.5.12   The sponsor should inform the investigator(s)/institution(s) in writing of the need for record retention and should notify the investigator(s)/institution(s) in writing when the trial related records are no longer needed.

5.6 Investigator Selection

5.6.1   The sponsor is responsible for selecting the investigator(s)/ institution(s). Each investigator should be qualified by training and experience and should have adequate resources (see 4.1, 4.2) to properly conduct the trial for which the investigator is selected. If organization of a coordinating committee and/or selection of coordinating investigator(s) are to be utilized in multicentre trials, their organization and/or selection are the sponsor's responsibility.

5.6.2   Before entering an agreement with an investigator/ institution to conduct a trial, the sponsor should provide the investigator(s)/institution(s) with the protocol and an up-to-date Investigator's Brochure, and should provide sufficient time for the investigator/institution to review the protocol and the information provided.

5.6.3   The sponsor should obtain the investigator's/institution's agreement:

(a) to conduct the trial in compliance with GCP, with the applicable regulatory requirement(s) (see 4.1.3), and with the protocol agreed to by the sponsor and given approval/favorable opinion by the IRB/IEC (see 4.5.1);

(b) to comply with procedures for data recording/reporting;

(c) to permit monitoring, auditing and inspection (see 4.1.4) and

(d) to retain the trial related essential documents until the sponsor informs the investigator/institution these documents are no longer needed (see 4.9.4 and 5.5.12).

The sponsor and the investigator/institution should sign the protocol, or an alternative document, to confirm this agreement.

5.7 Allocation of Responsibilities

Prior to initiating a trial, the sponsor should define, establish, and allocate all trial-related duties and functions.

5.8 Compensation to Subjects and Investigators

5.8.1   If required by the applicable regulatory requirement(s), the sponsor should provide insurance or should indemnify (legal and financial coverage) the investigator/the institution against claims arising from the trial, except for claims that arise from malpractice and/or negligence.

5.8.2   The sponsor's policies and procedures should address the costs of treatment of trial subjects in the event of trial-related injuries in accordance with the applicable regulatory requirement(s).

5.8.3   When trial subjects receive compensation, the method and manner of compensation should comply with applicable regulatory requirement(s).

5.9 Financing

The financial aspects of the trial should be documented in an agreement between the sponsor and the investigator/institution.

5.10 Notification/Submission to Regulatory Authority(ies)

Before initiating the clinical trial(s), the sponsor (or the sponsor and the investigator, if required by the applicable regulatory requirement(s)) should submit any required application(s) to the appropriate authority(ies) for review, acceptance, and/or permission (as required by the applicable regulatory requirement(s)) to begin the trial(s). Any notification/submission should be dated and contain sufficient information to identify the protocol.

5.11 Confirmation of Review by IRB/IEC

5.11.1   The sponsor should obtain from the investigator/institution:

(a) The name and address of the investigator's/institution's IRB/IEC.
(b) A statement obtained from the IRB/IEC that it is organized and operates according to GCP and the applicable laws and regulations.

(c) Documented IRB/IEC approval/favorable opinion and, if requested by the sponsor, a current copy of protocol, written informed consent form(s) and any other written information to be provided to subjects, subject recruiting procedures, and documents related to payments and compensation available to the subjects, and any other documents that the IRB/IEC may have requested.

5.11.2 If the IRB/IEC conditions its approval/favorable opinion upon change(s) in any aspect of the trial, such as modification(s) of the protocol, written informed consent form and any other written information to be provided to subjects, and/or other procedures, the sponsor should obtain from the investigator/ institution a copy of the modification(s) made and the date approval/favorable opinion was given by the IRB/IEC.

5.11.3 The sponsor should obtain from the investigator/institution documentation and dates of any IRB/IEC re-approvals/re-evaluations with favorable opinion, and of any withdrawals or suspensions of approval/favorable opinion.

5.12 Information on Investigational Product(s)

5.12.1 When planning trials, the sponsor should ensure that sufficient safety and efficacy data from nonclinical studies and/or clinical trials are available to support human exposure by the route, at the dosages, for the duration, and in the trial population to be studied.

5.12.2 The sponsor should update the Investigator's Brochure as significant new information becomes available (see 7. Investigator's Brochure).

5.13 Manufacturing, Packaging, Labeling, and Coding Investigational Product(s)

5.13.1 The sponsor should ensure that the investigational product(s) (including active comparator(s) and placebo, if applicable) is characterized as appropriate to the stage of development of the product(s), is manufactured in accordance with any applicable GMP, and is coded and labeled in a manner that protects the blinding, if applicable. In addition, the labeling should comply with applicable regulatory requirement(s).

5.13.2 The sponsor should determine, for the investigational product(s), acceptable storage temperatures, storage conditions (e.g., protection from light), storage times, reconstitution fluids and procedures, and devices for product infusion, if any. The sponsor should inform all involved parties (e.g., monitors, investigators, pharmacists, storage managers) of these determinations.

5.13.3 The investigational product(s) should be packaged to prevent contamination and unacceptable deterioration during transport and storage.

5.13.4 In blinded trials, the coding system for the investigational product(s) should include a mechanism that permits rapid identification of the product(s) in case of a medical emergency, but does not permit undetectable breaks of the blinding.

5.13.5 If significant formulation changes are made in the investigational or comparator product(s) during the course of clinical development, the results of any additional studies of the formulated product(s) (e.g., stability, dissolution rate, bioavailability) needed to assess whether these changes would significantly alter the pharmacokinetic profile of the product should be available prior to the use of the new formulation in clinical trials.

5.14 Supplying and Handling Investigational Product(s)

5.14.1   The sponsor is responsible for supplying the investigator(s)/ institution(s) with the investigational product(s).

5.14.2   The sponsor should not supply an investigator/institution with the investigational product(s) until the sponsor obtains all required documentation (e.g., approval/favorable opinion from IRB/IEC and regulatory authority(ies)).

5.14.3   The sponsor should ensure that written procedures include instructions that the investigator/institution should follow for the handling and storage of investigational product(s) for the trial and documentation thereof. The procedures should address adequate and safe receipt, handling, storage, dispensing, retrieval of unused product from subjects, and return of unused investigational product(s) to the sponsor (or alternative disposition if authorized by the sponsor and in compliance with the applicable regulatory requirement(s)).

5.14.4   The sponsor should:

   (a)   Ensure timely delivery of investigational product(s) to the investigator(s).
   (b)   Maintain records that document shipment, receipt, disposition, return, and destruction of the investigational product(s) (see 8. Essential Documents for the Conduct of a Clinical Trial).
   (c)   Maintain a system for retrieving investigational products and documenting this retrieval (e.g., for deficient product recall, reclaim after trial completion, expired product reclaim).
   (d)   Maintain a system for the disposition of unused investigational product(s) and for the documentation of this disposition.

5.14.5   The sponsor should:

   (a)   Take steps to ensure that the investigational product(s) are stable over the period of use.

(b) Maintain sufficient quantities of the investigational product(s) used in the trials to reconfirm specifications, should this become necessary, and maintain records of batch sample analyses and characteristics. To the extent stability permits, samples should be retained either until the analyses of the trial data are complete or as required by the applicable regulatory requirement(s), whichever represents the longer retention period.

5.15 Record Access

5.15.1 The sponsor should ensure that it is specified in the protocol or other written agreement that the investigator(s)/institution(s) provide direct access to source data/documents for trial-related monitoring, audits, IRB/IEC review, and regulatory inspection.

5.15.2 The sponsor should verify that each subject has consented, in writing, to direct access to his/her original medical records for trial-related monitoring, audit, IRB/IEC review, and regulatory inspection.

5.16 Safety Information

5.16.1 The sponsor is responsible for the ongoing safety evaluation of the investigational product(s).

5.16.2 The sponsor should promptly notify all concerned investigator(s)/institution(s) and the regulatory authority(ies) of findings that could affect adversely the safety of subjects, impact the conduct of the trial, or alter the IRB/IEC's approval/favorable opinion to continue the trial.

5.17 Adverse Drug Reaction Reporting

5.17.1 The sponsor should expedite the reporting to all concerned investigator(s)/institutions(s), to the IRB(s)/IEC(s), where required, and to the regulatory authority(ies) of all adverse drug reactions (ADRs) that are both serious and unexpected.

5.17.2　Such expedited reports should comply with the applicable regulatory requirement(s) and with the ICH Guideline for Clinical Safety Data Management: Definitions and Standards for Expedited Reporting.

5.17.3　The sponsor should submit to the regulatory authority(ies) all safety updates and periodic reports, as required by applicable regulatory requirement(s).

5.18　Monitoring

5.18.1　*Purpose*

The purposes of trial monitoring are to verify that:

(a)　The rights and well-being of human subjects are protected.
(b)　The reported trial data are accurate, complete, and verifiable from source documents.
(c)　The conduct of the trial is in compliance with the currently approved protocol/amendment(s), with GCP, and with the applicable regulatory requirement(s).

5.18.2　*Selection and Qualifications of Monitors*

(a)　Monitors should be appointed by the sponsor.
(b)　Monitors should be appropriately trained, and should have the scientific and/or clinical knowledge needed to monitor the trial adequately. A monitor's qualifications should be documented.
(c)　Monitors should be thoroughly familiar with the investigational product(s), the protocol, written informed consent form and any other written information to be provided to subjects, the sponsor's SOPs, GCP, and the applicable regulatory requirement(s).

5.18.3　*Extent and Nature of Monitoring*

The sponsor should ensure that the trials are adequately monitored. The sponsor should determine the appropriate extent and nature of monitoring. The determination of the extent and nature of monitoring should be based on considerations such as the objective, purpose, design, complexity, blinding, size, and endpoints of the trial. In general there is a need for on-site monitoring, before, during, and after the trial; however in exceptional circumstances the sponsor may determine that central monitoring in conjunction with procedures such as investigators' training and meetings, and extensive written guidance can assure appropriate conduct of the trial in accordance with GCP. Statistically controlled sampling may be an acceptable method for selecting the data to be verified.

ADDENDUM

The sponsor should develop a systematic, prioritized, risk-based approach to monitoring clinical trials. The flexibility in the extent and nature of monitoring described in this section is intended to permit varied approaches that improve the effectiveness and efficiency of monitoring. The sponsor may choose on-site monitoring, a combination of on-site and centralized monitoring, or, where justified, centralized monitoring. The sponsor should document the rationale for the chosen monitoring strategy (e.g., in the monitoring plan).

On-site monitoring is performed at the sites at which the clinical trial is being conducted. Centralized monitoring is a remote evaluation of accumulating data, performed in a timely manner, supported by appropriately qualified and trained persons (e.g., data managers, biostatisticians).

Centralized monitoring processes provide additional monitoring capabilities that can complement and reduce the extent and/or frequency of on-site monitoring and help distinguish between reliable data and potentially unreliable data.

Review that may include statistical analyses, of accumulating data from centralized monitoring can be used to:

(a) identify missing data, inconsistent data, data outliers, unexpected lack of variability and protocol deviations.

(b) examine data trends such as the range, consistency, and variability of data within and across sites.

(c) evaluate for systematic or significant errors in data collection and reporting at a site or across sites; or potential data manipulation or data integrity problems.

(d) analyze site characteristics and performance metrics.

(e) select sites and/or processes for targeted on-site monitoring.

5.18.4 Monitor's Responsibilities

The monitor(s) in accordance with the sponsor's requirements should ensure that the trial is conducted and documented properly by carrying out the following activities when relevant and necessary to the trial and the trial site:

(a) Acting as the main line of communication between the sponsor and the investigator.

(b) Verifying that the investigator has adequate qualifications and resources (see 4.1, 4.2, 5.6) and remain adequate throughout the trial period, that facilities, including laboratories, equipment, and staff, are adequate to safely and properly conduct the trial and remain adequate throughout the trial period.

(c) Verifying, for the investigational product(s):

(i) That storage times and conditions are acceptable, and that supplies are sufficient throughout the trial.

(ii) That the investigational product(s) are supplied only to subjects who are eligible to receive it and at the protocol specified dose(s).

(iii) That subjects are provided with necessary instruction on properly using, handling, storing, and returning the investigational product(s).

(iv) That the receipt, use, and return of the investigational product(s) at the trial sites are controlled and documented adequately.

(v) That the disposition of unused investigational product(s) at the trial sites complies with applicable regulatory requirement(s) and is in accordance with the sponsor.

(d) Verifying that the investigator follows the approved protocol and all approved amendment(s), if any.

(e) Verifying that written informed consent was obtained before each subject's participation in the trial.

(f) Ensuring that the investigator receives the current Investigator's Brochure, all documents, and all trial supplies needed to conduct the trial properly and to comply with the applicable regulatory requirement(s).

(g) Ensuring that the investigator and the investigator's trial staff are adequately informed about the trial.

(h) Verifying that the investigator and the investigator's trial staff are performing the specified trial functions, in accordance with the protocol and any other written agreement between the sponsor and the investigator/ institution, and have not delegated these functions to unauthorized individuals.

(i) Verifying that the investigator is enrolling only eligible subjects.

(j) Reporting the subject recruitment rate.

(k) Verifying that source documents and other trial records are accurate, complete, kept up-to-date and maintained.

(l) Verifying that the investigator provides all the required reports, notifications, applications, and submissions, and that these documents are accurate, complete, timely, legible, dated, and identify the trial.

(m) Checking the accuracy and completeness of the CRF entries, source documents and other trial-related records against each other. The monitor specifically should verify that:

(i) The data required by the protocol are reported accurately on the CRFs and are consistent with the source documents.

(ii) Any dose and/or therapy modifications are well documented for each of the trial subjects.

(iii) Adverse events, concomitant medications and intercurrent illnesses are reported in accordance with the protocol on the CRFs.

(iv) Visits that the subjects fail to make, tests that are not conducted, and examinations that are not performed are clearly reported as such on the CRFs.

(v) All withdrawals and dropouts of enrolled subjects from the trial are reported and explained on the CRFs.

(n) Informing the investigator of any CRF entry error, omission, or illegibility. The monitor should ensure that appropriate corrections, additions, or deletions are made, dated, explained (if necessary), and initialed by the investigator or by a member of the investigator's trial staff who is authorized to initial CRF changes for the investigator. This authorization should be documented.

(o) Determining whether all adverse events (AEs) are appropriately reported within the time periods required by GCP, the protocol, the IRB/IEC, the sponsor, and the applicable regulatory requirement(s).

(p) Determining whether the investigator is maintaining the essential documents (see 8. Essential Documents for the Conduct of a Clinical Trial).

(q) Communicating deviations from the protocol, SOPs, GCP, and the applicable regulatory requirements to the investigator and taking appropriate action designed to prevent recurrence of the detected deviations.

5.18.5   *Monitoring Procedures*

The monitor(s) should follow the sponsor's established written SOPs as well as those procedures that are specified by the sponsor for monitoring a specific trial.

5.18.6   *Monitoring Report*

(a) The monitor should submit a written report to the sponsor after each trial-site visit or trial-related communication.

(b) Reports should include the date, site, name of the monitor, and name of the investigator or other individual(s) contacted.

(c) Reports should include a summary of what the monitor reviewed and the monitor's statements concerning the significant findings/facts, deviations and deficiencies, conclusions, actions taken or to be taken and/or actions recommended to secure compliance.

(d) The review and follow-up of the monitoring report with the sponsor should be documented by the sponsor's designated representative.

ADDENDUM

(e) Reports of on-site and/or centralized monitoring should be provided to the sponsor (including appropriate management and staff responsible for trial and site oversight) in a timely manner for review and follow up. Results of monitoring activities should be documented in sufficient detail to allow verification of compliance with the monitoring plan. Reporting of centralized monitoring activities should be regular and may be independent from site visits.

ADDENDUM

5.18.7   *Monitoring Plan*

The sponsor should develop a monitoring plan that is tailored to the specific human subject protection and data integrity risks of the trial. The plan should describe the monitoring strategy, the monitoring responsibilities of all the parties involved, the various monitoring methods to be used, and the rationale for their use. The plan should also emphasize the monitoring of critical data and processes. Particular attention should be given to those aspects that are not routine clinical practice and that require additional training. The monitoring plan should reference the applicable policies and procedures.

5.19 Audit

If or when sponsors perform audits, as part of implementing quality assurance, they should consider:

5.19.1 *Purpose*

The purpose of a sponsor's audit, which is independent of and separate from routine monitoring or quality control functions, should be to evaluate trial conduct and compliance with the protocol, SOPs, GCP, and the applicable regulatory requirements.

5.19.2 *Selection and Qualification of Auditors*

(a) The sponsor should appoint individuals, who are independent of the clinical trials/systems, to conduct audits.

(b) The sponsor should ensure that the auditors are qualified by training and experience to conduct audits properly. An auditor's qualifications should be documented.

5.19.3 *Auditing Procedures*

(a) The sponsor should ensure that the auditing of clinical trials/systems is conducted in accordance with the sponsor's written procedures on what to audit, how to audit, the frequency of audits, and the form and content of audit reports.

(b) The sponsor's audit plan and procedures for a trial audit should be guided by the importance of the trial to submissions to regulatory authorities, the number of subjects in the trial, the type and complexity of the trial, the level of risks to the trial subjects, and any identified problem(s).

(c) The observations and findings of the auditor(s) should be documented.

(d) To preserve the independence and value of the audit function, the regulatory authority(ies) should not routinely request the audit reports. Regulatory authority(ies) may seek access to an audit report on a case by case basis when evidence of serious GCP non-compliance exists, or in the course of legal proceedings.

(e) When required by applicable law or regulation, the sponsor should provide an audit certificate.

5.20   Noncompliance

5.20.1   Noncompliance with the protocol, SOPs, GCP, and/or applicable regulatory requirement(s) by an investigator/ institution, or by member(s) of the sponsor's staff should lead to prompt action by the sponsor to secure compliance.

ADDENDUM

If noncompliance that significantly affects or has the potential to significantly affect human subject protection or reliability of trial results is discovered, the sponsor should perform a root cause analysis and implement appropriate corrective and preventive actions.

5.20.2   If the monitoring and/or auditing identifies serious and/ or persistent noncompliance on the part of an investigator/ institution, the sponsor should terminate the investiga- tor's/ institution's participation in the trial. When an investigator's/ institution's parti- cipation is terminated because of noncompliance, the sponsor should notify promptly the regulatory authority(ies).

5.21   Premature Termination or Suspension of a Trial

If a trial is prematurely terminated or suspended, the sponsor should promptly inform the investigators/institutions, and the regulatory authority(ies) of the termination or suspension and the reason(s) for the termination or suspension. The IRB/IEC should also be informed promptly and provided the reason(s) for the termination or suspension by the sponsor or by the investigator/institution, as specified by the applicable regulatory requirement(s).

5.22 Clinical Trial/Study Reports

Whether the trial is completed or prematurely terminated, the sponsor should ensure that the clinical trial reports are prepared and provided to the regulatory agency(ies) as required by the applicable regulatory requirement(s). The sponsor should also ensure that the clinical trial reports in marketing applications meet the standards of the ICH Guideline for Structure and Content of

Clinical Study Reports. (NOTE: The ICH Guideline for Structure and Content of Clinical Study Reports specifies that abbreviated study reports may be acceptable in certain cases.)

5.23 Multicentre Trials

For multicentre trials, the sponsor should ensure that:

5.23.1 All investigators conduct the trial in strict compliance with the protocol agreed to by the sponsor and, if required, by the regulatory authority(ies), and given approval/favorable opinion by the IRB/IEC.

5.23.2 The CRFs are designed to capture the required data at all multicentre trial sites. For those investigators who are collecting additional data, supplemental CRFs should also be provided that are designed to capture the additional data.

5.23.3 The responsibilities of coordinating investigator(s) and the other participating investigators are documented prior to the start of the trial.

5.23.4 All investigators are given instructions on following the protocol, on complying with a uniform set of standards for the assessment of clinical and laboratory findings, and on completing the CRFs.

5.23.5 Communication between investigators is facilitated.

6.   CLINICAL TRIAL PROTOCOL AND PROTOCOL AMENDMENT(S)

The contents of a trial protocol should generally include the following topics. However, site specific information may be provided on separate protocol page(s), or addressed in a separate agreement, and some of the information listed below may be contained in other protocol referenced documents, such as an Investigator's Brochure.

6.1   General Information

6.1.1   Protocol title, protocol identifying number, and date. Any amendment(s) should also bear the amendment number(s) and date(s).

6.1.2   Name and address of the sponsor and monitor (if other than the sponsor).

6.1.3   Name and title of the person(s) authorized to sign the protocol and the protocol amendment(s) for the sponsor.

6.1.4   Name, title, address, and telephone number(s) of the sponsor's medical expert (or dentist when appropriate) for the trial.

6.1.5   Name and title of the investigator(s) who is (are) responsible for conducting the trial, and the address and telephone number(s) of the trial site(s).

6.1.6   Name, title, address, and telephone number(s) of the qualified physician (or dentist, if applicable), who is responsible for all trial-site related medical (or dental) decisions (if other than investigator).

6.1.7   Name(s) and address(es) of the clinical laboratory(ies) and other medical and/or technical department(s) and/or institutions involved in the trial.

6.2   Background Information

6.2.1   Name and description of the investigational product(s).

6.2.2   A summary of findings from nonclinical studies that potentially have clinical significance and from clinical trials that are relevant to the trial.

6.2.3   Summary of the known and potential risks and benefits, if any, to human subjects.

6.2.4   Description of and justification for the route of administration, dosage, dosage regimen, and treatment period(s).

6.2.5   A statement that the trial will be conducted in compliance with the protocol, GCP and the applicable regulatory requirement(s).

6.2.6   Description of the population to be studied.

6.2.7   References to literature and data that are relevant to the trial, and that provide background for the trial.

6.3   Trial Objectives and Purpose

A detailed description of the objectives and the purpose of the trial.

6.4   Trial Design

The scientific integrity of the trial and the credibility of the data from the trial depend substantially on the trial design. A description of the trial design, should include:

6.4.1   A specific statement of the primary endpoints and the secondary endpoints, if any, to be measured during the trial.

6.4.2   A description of the type/design of trial to be conducted (e.g., double-blind, placebo- controlled, parallel design) and a schematic diagram of trial design, procedures and stages.

6.4.3   A description of the measures taken to minimize/avoid bias, including:
(a)   Randomization.
(b)   Blinding.

6.4.4   A description of the trial treatment(s) and the dosage and dosage regimen of the investigational product(s). Also include a description of the dosage form, packaging, and labelling of the investigational product(s).

6.4.5   The expected duration of subject participation, and a description of the sequence and duration of all trial periods, including follow-up, if any.

6.4.6   A description of the "stopping rules" or "discontinuation criteria" for individual subjects, parts of trial and entire trial.

6.4.7   Accountability procedures for the investigational product(s), including the placebo(s) and comparator(s), if any.

6.4.8   Maintenance of trial treatment randomization codes and procedures for breaking codes.

6.4.9   The identification of any data to be recorded directly on the CRFs (i.e., no prior written or electronic record of data), and to be considered to be source data.

6.5   Selection and Withdrawal of Subjects

6.5.1   Subject inclusion criteria.

6.5.2   Subject exclusion criteria.

6.5.3   Subject withdrawal criteria (i.e., terminating investigational product treatment/trial treatment) and procedures specifying:

(a)   When and how to withdraw subjects from the trial/ investigational product treatment.
(b)   The type and timing of the data to be collected for withdrawn subjects.
(c)   Whether and how subjects are to be replaced.
(d)   The follow-up for subjects withdrawn from investigational product treatment/trial treatment.

6.6 Treatment of Subjects

6.6.1 The treatment(s) to be administered, including the name(s) of all the product(s), the dose(s), the dosing schedule(s), the route/mode(s) of administration, and the treatment period(s), including the follow-up period(s) for subjects for each investigational product treatment/trial treatment group/ arm of the trial.

6.6.2 Medication(s)/treatment(s) permitted (including rescue medication) and not permitted before and/or during the trial.

6.6.3 Procedures for monitoring subject compliance.

6.7 Assessment of Efficacy

6.7.1 Specification of the efficacy parameters.

6.7.2 Methods and timing for assessing, recording, and analyzing of efficacy parameters.

6.8 Assessment of Safety

6.8.1 Specification of safety parameters.

6.8.2 The methods and timing for assessing, recording, and analyzing safety parameters.

6.8.3 Procedures for eliciting reports of and for recording and reporting adverse event and intercurrent illnesses.

6.8.4 The type and duration of the follow-up of subjects after adverse events.

6.9 Statistics

6.9.1 A description of the statistical methods to be employed, including timing of any planned interim analysis(ses).

6.9.2 The number of subjects planned to be enrolled. In multicentre trials, the numbers of enrolled subjects projected for each trial site should be specified. Reason for choice of sample size, including reflections on (or calculations of) the power of the trial and clinical justification.

6.9.3   The level of significance to be used.

6.9.4   Criteria for the termination of the trial.

6.9.5   Procedure for accounting for missing, unused, and spurious data.

6.9.6   Procedures for reporting any deviation(s) from the original statistical plan (any deviation(s) from the original statistical plan should be described and justified in protocol and/or in the final report, as appropriate).

6.9.7   The selection of subjects to be included in the analyses (e.g., all randomized subjects, all dosed subjects, all eligible subjects, evaluable subjects).

6.10   Direct Access to Source Data/Documents

The sponsor should ensure that it is specified in the protocol or other written agreement that the investigator(s)/institution(s) will permit trial-related monitoring, audits, IRB/IEC review, and regulatory inspection(s), providing direct access to source data/documents.

6.11   Quality Control and Quality Assurance

6.12   Ethics

Description of ethical considerations relating to the trial.

6.13   Data Handling and Record Keeping

6.14   Financing and Insurance

Financing and insurance if not addressed in a separate agreement.

6.15   Publication Policy

Publication policy, if not addressed in a separate agreement.

6.16 Supplements

(NOTE: Since the protocol and the clinical trial/study report are closely related, further relevant information can be found in the ICH Guideline for Structure and Content of Clinical Study Reports.)

7. INVESTIGATOR'S BROCHURE

7.1 Introduction

The Investigator's Brochure (IB) is a compilation of the clinical and nonclinical data on the investigational product(s) that are relevant to the study of the product(s) in human subjects. Its purpose is to provide the investigators and others involved in the trial with the information to facilitate their understanding of the rationale for, and their compliance with, many key features of the protocol, such as the dose, dose frequency/interval, methods of administration: and safety monitoring procedures. The IB also provides insight to support the clinical management of the study subjects during the course of the clinical trial. The information should be presented in a concise, simple, objective, balanced, and non-promotional form that enables a clinician, or potential investigator, to understand it and make his/her own unbiased risk-benefit assessment of the appropriateness of the proposed trial. For this reason, a medically qualified person should generally participate in the editing of an IB, but the contents of the IB should be approved by the disciplines that generated the described data.

This guideline delineates the minimum information that should be included in an IB and provides suggestions for its layout. It is expected that the type and extent of information available will vary with the stage of development of the investigational product. If the investigational product is marketed and its pharmacology is widely understood by medical practitioners, an extensive IB may not be necessary. Where permitted by regulatory authorities, a basic product information brochure, package leaflet, or labelling may be an appropriate alternative, provided that it includes current, comprehensive, and detailed information on all aspects of the investigational product that might be of importance to the investigator. If a marketed product is being studied for a new use (i.e., a new indication), an IB specific to that new use should be prepared. The IB should be reviewed at least annually and revised as necessary in compliance with a sponsor's written procedures. More frequent revision may be appropriate depending on the stage of development and the generation of relevant new information. However, in accordance with Good Clinical Practice, relevant new information may be so important that it should be communicated to the investigators, and possibly to the Institutional Review Boards (IRBs)/Independent Ethics Committees (IECs) and/ or regulatory authorities before it is included in a revised IB.

Generally, the sponsor is responsible for ensuring that an up-to-date IB is made available to the investigator(s) and the investigators are responsible for providing the up-to-date IB to the responsible IRBs/ IECs. In the case of an investigator sponsored trial, the sponsor-investigator should determine whether a brochure is available from the commercial manufacturer. If the investigational product is provided by the sponsor-investigator, then he or she should provide the necessary information to the trial personnel. In cases where preparation of a formal IB is impractical, the sponsor-investigator should provide, as a substitute, an expanded background information section in the trial protocol that contains the minimum current information described in this guideline.

7.2 General Considerations

The IB should include:

7.2.1 Title Page

This should provide the sponsor's name, the identity of each investigational product (i.e., research number, chemical or approved generic name, and trade name(s) where legally permissible and desired by the sponsor), and the release date. It is also suggested that an edition number, and a reference to the number and date of the edition it supersedes, be provided. An example is given in Appendix 1.

7.2.2   *Confidentiality Statement*

The sponsor may wish to include a statement instructing the investigator/recipients to treat the IB as a confidential document for the sole information and use of the investigator's team and the IRB/IEC.

7.3   Contents of the Investigator's Brochure

The IB should contain the following sections, each with literature references where appropriate:

7.3.1   *Table of Contents*

An example of the Table of Contents is given in Appendix 2

7.3.2   *Summary*

A brief summary (preferably not exceeding two pages) should be given, highlighting the significant physical, chemical, pharmaceutical, pharmacological, toxicological, pharmacokinetic, metabolic, and clinical information available that is relevant to the stage of clinical development of the investigational product.

7.3.3   *Introduction*

A brief introductory statement should be provided that contains the chemical name (and generic and trade name(s) when approved) of the investigational product(s), all active ingredients, the investigational product (s) pharmacological class and its expected position within this class (e.g., advantages), the rationale for performing research with the investigational product(s), and the anticipated prophylactic, therapeutic, or diagnostic indication(s). Finally, the introductory statement should provide the general approach to be followed in evaluating the investigational product.

7.3.4   *Physical, Chemical, and Pharmaceutical Properties and Formulation*

A description should be provided of the investigational product substance(s) (including the chemical and/or structural formula(e)), and a brief summary should be given of the relevant physical, chemical, and pharmaceutical properties.

To permit appropriate safety measures to be taken in the course of the trial, a description of the formulation(s) to be used, including excipients, should be provided and justified if clinically relevant. Instructions for the storage and handling of the dosage form(s) should also be given.

Any structural similarities to other known compounds should be mentioned.

7.3.5 *Nonclinical Studies*

Introduction:

The results of all relevant nonclinical pharmacology, toxicology, pharmacokinetic, and investigational product metabolism studies should be provided in summary form. This summary should address the methodology used, the results, and a discussion of the relevance of the findings to the investigated therapeutic and the possible unfavourable and unintended effects in humans.

The information provided may include the following, as appropriate, if known/available:

- Species tested
- Number and sex of animals in each group
- Unit dose (e.g., milligram/kilogram (mg/kg))
- Dose interval
- Route of administration
- Duration of dosing
- Information on systemic distribution
- Duration of post-exposure follow-up
- Results, including the following aspects:
    - Nature and frequency of pharmacological or toxic effects
    - Severity or intensity of pharmacological or toxic effects
    - Time to onset of effects
    - Reversibility of effects
    - Duration of effects
    - Dose response

Tabular format/listings should be used whenever possible to enhance the clarity of the presentation.

The following sections should discuss the most important findings from the studies, including the dose response of observed effects, the relevance to humans, and any aspects to be studied in humans. If applicable, the effective and nontoxic dose findings in the same animal species should be compared (i.e., the therapeutic index should be discussed). The relevance of this information to the proposed human dosing should be addressed. Whenever possible, comparisons should be made in terms of blood/tissue levels rather than on a mg/kg basis.

(a) Nonclinical Pharmacology

A summary of the pharmacological aspects of the investigational product and, where appropriate, its significant metabolites studied in animals, should be included. Such a summary should incorporate studies that assess potential therapeutic activity (e.g., efficacy models, receptor binding, and specificity) as well as those that assess safety (e.g., special studies to assess pharmacological actions other than the intended therapeutic effect(s)).

(b) Pharmacokinetics and Product Metabolism in Animals

A summary of the pharmacokinetics and biological transformation and disposition of the investigational product in all species studied should be given. The discussion of the findings should address the absorption and the local and systemic bioavailability of the investigational product and its metabolites, and their relationship to the pharmacological and toxicological findings in animal species.

(c) Toxicology

A summary of the toxicological effects found in relevant studies conducted in different animal species should be described under the following headings where appropriate:

- Single dose
- Repeated dose
- Carcinogenicity
- Special studies (e.g., irritancy and sensitisation)
- Reproductive toxicity
- Genotoxicity (mutagenicity)

7.3.6   Effects in Humans

Introduction:

A thorough discussion of the known effects of the investigational product(s) in humans should be provided, including information on pharmacokinetics, metabolism, pharmacodynamics, dose response, safety, efficacy, and other pharmacological activities. Where possible, a summary of each completed clinical trial should be provided. Information should also be provided regarding results of any use of the investigational product(s) other than from in clinical trials, such as from experience during marketing.

(a) Pharmacokinetics and Product Metabolism in Humans

- A summary of information on the pharmacokinetics of the investigational product(s) should be presented, including the following, if available:
- Pharmacokinetics (including metabolism, as appropriate, and absorption, plasma protein binding, distribution, and elimination).
- Bioavailability of the investigational product (absolute, where possible, and/or relative) using a reference dosage form.
- Population subgroups (e.g., gender, age, and impaired organ function).
- Interactions (e.g., product-product interactions and effects of food).
- Other pharmacokinetic data (e.g., results of population studies performed within clinical trial(s).

(b) Safety and Efficacy

A summary of information should be provided about the investigational product's/products' (including metabolites, where appropriate) safety, pharmacodynamics, efficacy, and dose response that were obtained from preceding trials in humans (healthy volunteers and/or patients). The implications of this information should be discussed. In cases where a number of clinical trials have been completed, the use of summaries of safety and efficacy across multiple trials by indications in subgroups may provide a clear presentation of the data. Tabular summaries of adverse drug reactions for all the clinical trials (including those for all the studied indications) would be useful. Important differences in adverse drug reaction patterns/incidences across indications or subgroups should be discussed.

The IB should provide a description of the possible risks and adverse drug reactions to be anticipated on the basis of prior experiences with the product under investigation and with related products. A description should also be provided of the precautions or special monitoring to be done as part of the investigational use of the product(s).

(c) Marketing Experience

The IB should identify countries where the investigational product has been marketed or approved. Any significant information arising from the marketed use should be summarised (e.g., formulations, dosages, routes of administration, and adverse product reactions). The IB should also identify all the countries where the investigational product did not receive approval/registration for marketing or was withdrawn from marketing/registration.

7.3.7   Summary of Data and Guidance for the Investigator

This section should provide an overall discussion of the nonclinical and clinical data, and should summarise the information from various sources on different aspects of the investigational product(s), wherever possible. In this way, the investigator can be provided with the most informative interpretation of the available data and with an assessment of the implications of the information for future clinical trials.

Where appropriate, the published reports on related products should be discussed. This could help the investigator to anticipate adverse drug reactions or other problems in clinical trials.

The overall aim of this section is to provide the investigator with a clear understanding of the possible risks and adverse reactions, and of the specific tests, observations, and precautions that may be needed for a clinical trial. This understanding should be based on the available physical, chemical, pharmaceutical, pharmacological, toxicological, and clinical information on the investigational product(s). Guidance should also be provided to the clinical investigator on the recognition and treatment of possible overdose and adverse drug reactions that is based on previous human experience and on the pharmacology of the investigational product.

7.4   APPENDIX 1:

TITLE PAGE *(Example)*
SPONSOR'S NAME
   Product:
   Research Number:
   Name(s):   Chemical, Generic (if approved)
            Trade Name(s) (if legally permissible and desired by
            the sponsor)

INVESTIGATOR'S
BROCHURE

Edition Number:
Release Date:

Replaces Previous Edition Number:
Date:

7.5 APPENDIX 2:

TABLE OF CONTENTS OF INVESTIGATOR'S BROCHURE
(Example)

NB: References on   1. Publications

2. Reports

These references should be found at the end of each chapter
Appendices (if any)

8. ESSENTIAL DOCUMENTS FOR THE CONDUCT OF A CLINICAL TRIAL

8.1 Introduction

Essential Documents are those documents which individually and collectively permit evaluation of the conduct of a trial and the quality of the data produced. These documents serve to demonstrate the compliance of the investigator, sponsor and monitor with the standards of Good Clinical Practice and with all applicable regulatory requirements.

Essential Documents also serve a number of other important purposes. Filing essential documents at the investigator/institution and sponsor sites in a timely manner can greatly assist in the successful management of a trial by the investigator, sponsor and monitor. These documents are also the ones which are usually audited by the sponsor's independent audit function and inspected by the regulatory authority(ies) as part of the process to confirm the validity of the trial conduct and the integrity of data collected.

The minimum list of essential documents which has been developed follows. The various documents are grouped in three sections according to the stage of the trial during which they will normally be generated: 1) before the clinical phase of the trial commences, 2) during the clinical conduct of the trial, and 3) after completion or termination of the trial. A description is given of the purpose of each document, and whether it should be filed in either the investigator/institution or sponsor files, or both. It is acceptable to combine some of the documents, provided the individual elements are readily identifiable.

Trial master files should be established at the beginning of the trial, both at the investigator/institution's site and at the sponsor's office. A final close-out of a trial can only be done when the monitor has reviewed both investigator/institution and sponsor files and confirmed that all necessary documents are in the appropriate files.

Any or all of the documents addressed in this guideline may be subject to, and should be available for, audit by the sponsor's auditor and inspection by the regulatory authority(ies).

ADDENDUM

The sponsor and investigator/institution should maintain a record of the location(s) of their respective essential documents including source documents. The storage system used during the trial and for archiving (irrespective of the type of media used) should provide for document identification, version history, search, and retrieval.

Essential documents for the trial should be supplemented or may be reduced where justified (in advance of trial initiation) based on the importance and relevance of the specific documents to the trial.

The sponsor should ensure that the investigator has control of and continuous access to the CRF data reported to the sponsor. The sponsor should not have exclusive control of those data.

When a copy is used to replace an original document (e.g., source documents, CRF), the copy should fulfill the requirements for certified copies.

The investigator/institution should have control of all essential documents and records generated by the investigator/institution before, during, and after the trial.

8.2 Before the Clinical Phase of the Trial Commences

During this planning stage the following documents should be generated and should be on file before the trial formally starts

	Title of Document	Purpose	Located in Files of	
			Investigator/ Institution	Sponsor
8.2.1	**INVESTIGATOR'S BROCHURE**	To document that relevant and current scientific information about the investigational product has been provided to the investigator	X	X
8.2.2	**SIGNED PROTOCOL AND AMENDMENTS, IF ANY, AND SAMPLE CASE REPORT FORM (CRF)**	To document investigator and sponsor agreement to the protocol/amendment(s) and CRF	X	X
8.2.3	**INFORMATION GIVEN TO TRIAL SUBJECT** **- INFORMED CONSENT FORM** (including all applicable translations)	To document the informed consent	X	X
	- ANY OTHER WRITTEN INFORMATION	To document that subjects will be given appropriate written information (content and wording) to support their ability to give fully informed consent	X	X

	Title of Document	Purpose	Located in Files of	
			Investigator/ Institution	Sponsor
	- ADVERTISEMENT FOR SUBJECT RECRUITMENT (if used)	To document that recruitment measures are appropriate and not coercive	X	
8.2.4	**FINANCIAL ASPECTS OF THE TRIAL**	To document the financial agreement between the investigator/institution and the sponsor for the trial	X	X
8.2.5	**INSURANCE STATEMENT** (where required)	To document that compensation to subject(s) for trial-related injury will be available	X	X
8.2.6	**SIGNED AGREEMENT BETWEEN INVOLVED PARTIES**, e.g.: - investigator/institution and sponsor - investigator/institution and CRO - sponsor and CRO - investigator/institution and authority(ies) (where required)	To document agreements	X X X	X X (where required) X X

	Title of Document	Purpose	Located in Files of	
			Investigator/ Institution	Sponsor
8.2.7	**DATED, DOCUMENTED APPROVAL/ FAVOURABLE OPINION OF INSTITUTIONAL REVIEW BOARD (IRB) /INDEPENDENT ETHICS COMMITTEE (IEC) OF THE FOLLOWING:** - protocol and any amendments - CRF (if applicable) - informed consent form(s) - any other written information to be provided to the subject(s) - advertisement for subject recruitment (if used) - subject compensation (if any) - any other documents given approval/ favourable opinion	To document that the trial has been subject to IRB/IEC review and given approval/ favourable opinion. To identify the version number and date of the document(s)	X	X
8.2.8	**INSTITUTIONAL REVIEW BOARD/ INDEPENDENT ETHICS COMMITTEE COMPOSITION**	To document that the IRB/IEC is constituted in agreement with GCP	X	X (where required)

	Title of Document	Purpose	Located in Files of	
			Investigator/ Institution	Sponsor
8.2.9	**REGULATORY AUTHORITY(IES) AUTHORISATION/APPROVAL/ NOTIFICATION OF PROTOCOL** (where required)	To document appropriate authorisation/ approval/notification by the regulatory authority(ies) has been obtained prior to initiation of the trial in compliance with the applicable regulatory requirement(s)	X (where required)	X (where required)
8.2.10	**CURRICULUM VITAE AND/OR OTHER RELEVANT DOCUMENTS EVIDENCING QUALIFICATIONS OF INVESTIGATOR(S) AND SUB-INVESTIGATOR(S)**	To document qualifications and eligibility to conduct trial and/or provide medical supervision of subjects	X	X
8.2.11	**NORMAL VALUE(S)/RANGE(S) FOR MEDICAL/ LABORATORY/TECHNICAL PROCEDURE(S) AND/OR TEST(S) INCLUDED IN THE PROTOCOL**	To document normal values and/or ranges of the tests	X	X

	Title of Document	Purpose	Located in Files of	
			Investigator/ Institution	Sponsor
8.2.12	MEDICAL/LABORATORY/TECHNICAL PROCEDURES /TESTS - certification or - accreditation or - established quality control and/or external quality assessment or - other validation (where required)	To document competence of facility to perform required test(s), and support reliability of results	X (where required)	X
8.2.13	SAMPLE OF LABEL(S) ATTACHED TO INVESTIGATIONAL PRODUCT CONTAINER(S)	To document compliance with applicable labelling regulations and appropriateness of instructions provided to the subjects		X
8.2.14	INSTRUCTIONS FOR HANDLING OF INVESTIGATIONAL PRODUCT(S) AND TRIAL-RELATED MATERIALS (if not included in protocol or Investigator's Brochure)	To document instructions needed to ensure proper storage, packaging, dispensing and disposition of investigational products and trial-related materials	X	X
8.2.15	SHIPPING RECORDS FOR INVESTIGATIONAL PRODUCT(S) AND TRIAL-RELATED MATERIALS	To document shipment dates, batch numbers and method of shipment of investigational product(s) and trial-related materials. Allows tracking of product batch, review of shipping conditions, and accountability	X	X

	Title of Document	Purpose	Located in Files of	
			Investigator/ Institution	Sponsor
8.2.16	CERTIFICATE(S) OF ANALYSIS OF INVESTIGATIONAL PRODUCT(S) SHIPPED	To document identity, purity, and strength of investigational product(s) to be used in the trial		X
8.2.17	DECODING PROCEDURES FOR BLINDED TRIALS	To document how, in case of an emergency, identity of blinded investigational product can be revealed without breaking the blind for the remaining subjects' treatment	X	X (third party if applicable)
8.2.18	MASTER RANDOMISATION LIST	To document method for randomisation of trial population		X (third party if applicable)
8.2.19	PRE-TRIAL MONITORING REPORT	To document that the site is suitable for the trial (may be combined with 8.2.20)		X
8.2.20	TRIAL INITIATION MONITORING REPORT	To document that trial procedures were reviewed with the investigator and the investigator's trial staff (may be combined with 8.2.19)	X	X

8.3 During the Clinical Conduct of the Trial

In addition to having on file the above documents, the following should be added to the files during the trial as evidence that all new relevant information is documented as it becomes available

	Title of Document	Purpose	Located in Files of	
			Investigator/ Institution	Sponsor
8.3.1	**INVESTIGATOR'S BROCHURE UPDATES**	To document that investigator is informed in a timely manner of relevant information as it becomes available	X	X
8.3.2	**ANY REVISION TO:** - protocol/amendment(s) and CRF - informed consent form - any other written information provided to subjects - advertisement for subject recruitment (if used)	To document revisions of these trial related documents that take effect during trial	X	X

	Title of Document	Purpose	Located in Files of	
			Investigator/ Institution	Sponsor

8.3.3	DATED, DOCUMENTED APPROVAL/ FAVOURABLE OPINION OF INSTITUTIONAL REVIEW BOARD (IRB) /INDEPENDENT ETHICS COMMITTEE (IEC) OF THE FOLLOWING:
	- protocol amendment(s)
	- revision(s) of:
	  - informed consent form
	  - any other written information to be provided to the subject
	  - advertisement for subject recruitment (if used)
	- any other documents given approval/ favourable opinion
	- continuing review of trial (where required)
		To document that the amendment(s) and/ or revision(s) have been subject to IRB/IEC review and were given approval/favourable opinion. To identify the version number and date of the document(s).	X	X

8.3.4	REGULATORY AUTHORITY(IES) AUTHORISATIONS/APPROVALS/ NOTIFICATIONS WHERE REQUIRED FOR: - protocol amendment(s) and other documents	To document compliance with applicable regulatory requirements	X (where required)	X

	Title of Document	Purpose	Located in Files of	
			Investigator/ Institution	Sponsor
8.3.5	**CURRICULUM VITAE FOR NEW INVESTIGATOR(S) AND/OR SUB- INVESTIGATOR(S)**	(see 8.2.10)	X	X
8.3.6	**UPDATES TO NORMAL VALUE(S)/ RANGE(S) FOR MEDICAL/ LABORATORY/ TECHNICAL PROCEDURE(S)/TEST(S) INCLUDED IN THE PROTOCOL**	To document normal values and ranges that are revised during the trial (see 8.2.11)	X	X
8.3.7	**UPDATES OF MEDICAL/LABORATORY/ TECHNICAL PROCEDURES/TESTS** - certification or - accreditation or - established quality control and/or external quality assessment or - other validation (where required)	To document that tests remain adequate throughout the trial period (see 8.2.12)	X (where required)	X
8.3.8	**DOCUMENTATION OF INVESTIGATIONAL PRODUCT(S) AND TRIAL-RELATED MATERIALS SHIPMENT**	(see 8.2.15.)	X	X

	Title of Document	Purpose	Located in Files of	
			Investigator/ Institution	Sponsor
8.3.9	**CERTIFICATE(S) OF ANALYSIS FOR NEW BATCHES OF INVESTIGATIONAL PRODUCTS**	(see 8.2.16)		X
8.3.10	**MONITORING VISIT REPORTS**	To document site visits by, and findings of, the monitor		X
8.3.11	**RELEVANT COMMUNICATIONS OTHER THAN SITE VISITS** - letters - meeting notes - notes of telephone calls	To document any agreements or significant discussions regarding trial administration, protocol violations, trial conduct, adverse event (AE) reporting	X	X
8.3.12	**SIGNED INFORMED CONSENT FORMS**	To document that consent is obtained in accordance with GCP and protocol and dated prior to participation of each subject in trial. Also to document direct access permission (see 8.2.3)	X	
8.3.13	**SOURCE DOCUMENTS**	To document the existence of the subject and substantiate integrity of trial data collected. To include original documents related to the trial, to medical treatment, and history of subject	X	

	Title of Document	Purpose	Located in Files of	
			Investigator/ Institution	Sponsor
8.3.14	SIGNED, DATED AND COMPLETED CASE REPORT FORMS (CRF)	To document that the investigator or authorised member of the investigator's staff confirms the observations recorded	X (copy)	X (original)
8.3.15	DOCUMENTATION OF CRF CORRECTIONS	To document all changes/additions or corrections made to CRF after initial data were recorded	X (copy)	X (original)
8.3.16	NOTIFICATION BY ORIGINATING INVESTIGATOR TO SPONSOR OF SERIOUS ADVERSE EVENTS AND RELATED REPORTS	Notification by originating investigator to sponsor of serious adverse events and related reports in accordance with 4.11	X	X
8.3.17	NOTIFICATION BY SPONSOR AND/OR INVESTIGATOR, WHERE APPLICABLE, TO REGULATORY AUTHORITY(IES) AND IRB(S)/IEC(S) OF UNEXPECTED SERIOUS ADVERSE DRUG REACTIONS AND OF OTHER SAFETY INFORMATION	Notification by sponsor and/or investigator, where applicable, to regulatory authorities and IRB(s)/IEC(s) of unexpected serious adverse drug reactions in accordance with 5.17 and 4.11.1 and of other safety information in accordance with 5.16.2 and 4.11.2	X (where required)	X

	Title of Document	Purpose	Located in Files of Investigator/ Institution	Located in Files of Sponsor
8.3.18	**NOTIFICATION BY SPONSOR TO INVESTIGATORS OF SAFETY INFORMATION**	Notification by sponsor to investigators of safety information in accordance with 5.16.2	X	X
8.3.19	**INTERIM OR ANNUAL REPORTS TO IRB/IEC AND AUTHORITY(IES)**	Interim or annual reports provided to IRB/IEC in accordance with 4.10 and to authority(ies) in accordance with 5.17.3	X	X (where required)
8.3.20	**SUBJECT SCREENING LOG**	To document identification of subjects who entered pre-trial screening	X	X (where required)
8.3.21	**SUBJECT IDENTIFICATION CODE LIST**	To document that investigator/institution keeps a confidential list of names of all subjects allocated to trial numbers on enrolling in the trial. Allows investigator/ institution to reveal identity of any subject	X	
8.3.22	**SUBJECT ENROLMENT LOG**	To document chronological enrolment of subjects by trial number	X	
8.3.23	**INVESTIGATIONAL PRODUCTS ACCOUNTABILITY AT THE SITE**	To document that investigational product(s) have been used according to the protocol	X	X

	Title of Document	Purpose	Located in Files of	
			Investigator/ Institution	Sponsor
8.3.24	**SIGNATURE SHEET**	To document signatures and initials of all persons authorised to make entries and/or corrections on CRFs	X	X
8.3.25	**RECORD OF RETAINED BODY FLUIDS/ TISSUE SAMPLES (IF ANY)**	To document location and identification of retained samples if assays need to be repeated	X	X

8.4 After Completion or Termination of the Trial

After completion or termination of the trial, all of the documents identified in Sections 8.2 and 8.3 should be in the file together with the following

	Title of Document	Purpose	Located in Files of Investigator/Institution	Located in Files of Sponsor
8.4.1	INVESTIGATIONAL PRODUCT(S) ACCOUNTABILITY AT SITE	To document that the investigational product(s) have been used according to the protocol. To documents the final accounting of investigational product(s) received at the site, dispensed to subjects, returned by the subjects, and returned to sponsor	X	X
8.4.2	DOCUMENTATION OF INVESTIGATIONAL PRODUCT DESTRUCTION	To document destruction of unused investigational products by sponsor or at site	X (if destroyed at site)	X
8.4.3	COMPLETED SUBJECT IDENTIFICATION CODE LIST	To permit identification of all subjects enrolled in the trial in case follow-up is required. List should be kept in a confidential manner and for agreed upon time	X	
8.4.4	AUDIT CERTIFICATE (if available)	To document that audit was performed		X

	Title of Document	Purpose	Located in Files of Investigator/Institution	Located in Files of Sponsor
8.4.5	**FINAL TRIAL CLOSE-OUT MONITORING REPORT**	To document that all activities required for trial close-out are completed, and copies of essential documents are held in the appropriate files		X
8.4.6	**TREATMENT ALLOCATION AND DECODING DOCUMENTATION**	Returned to sponsor to document any decoding that may have occurred		X
8.4.7	**FINAL REPORT BY INVESTIGATOR TO IRB/IEC WHERE REQUIRED, AND WHERE APPLICABLE, TO THE REGULATORY AUTHORITY(IES)**	To document completion of the trial	X	
8.4.8	**CLINICAL STUDY REPORT**	To document results and interpretation of trial	X (if applicable)	X

INTERNATIONAL COUNCIL FOR HARMONISATION OF TECHNICAL
REQUIREMENTS FOR PHARMACEUTICALS FOR HUMAN USE

ICH HARMONISED GUIDELINE

GENERAL CONSIDERATIONS
FOR CLINICAL STUDIES

E8(R1)

Final version

Adopted on 6 October 2021

*This Guideline has been developed by the appropriate ICH Expert
Working Group and has been subject to consultation by the regulatory
parties, in accordance with the ICH Process. At Step 4 of the Process
the final draft is recommended for adoption to the regulatory bodies of
ICH regions.*

E8(R1)
Document

History E8

Code	History	Date
E8	Approval by the Steering Committee under *Step 4* and recommendation for adoption by ICH regulatory bodies.	17 July 1997

Revision of E8

Code	History	Date
E8(R1)	Adoption by the Regulatory Members of the ICH Assembly under *Step 4*.	6 October 2021
E8(R1)	Editorial correction approved by the MC under Section 5.6, 4th paragraph, page 16: addition of the word "plan".	4 February 2022

ICH HARMONISED GUIDELINE

GENERAL CONSIDERATIONS FOR CLINICAL STUDIES

E8(R1)

ICH Consensus Guideline

1. OBJECTIVES OF THIS DOCUMENT

Clinical studies of medicinal products are conducted to provide information that can ultimately improve access to safe and effective products with meaningful impact on patients, while protecting those participating in the studies. This document provides guidance on the clinical development lifecycle, including designing quality into clinical studies, considering the broad range of clinical study designs and data sources used.

The ICH document "General Considerations for Clinical Studies" is intended to:

1. Describe internationally accepted principles and practices in the design and conduct of clinical studies that will ensure the protection of study participants and facilitate acceptance of data and results by regulatory authorities
2. Provide guidance on the consideration of quality in the design and conduct of clinical studies across the product lifecycle, including the identification, during study planning, of factors that are critical to the quality of the study, and the management of risks to those factors during study conduct
3. Provide an overview of the types of clinical studies performed during the product lifecycle, and describe study design elements that support the identification of quality factors critical to ensuring the protection of study participants, the integrity of the data, the reliability of results, and the ability of the studies to meet their objectives
4. Provide a guide to the ICH efficacy documents to facilitate user's access

General principles are described in Section 2 of this document, followed by a discussion of designing quality into clinical studies in Section 3. A broad overview of drug development planning and the information provided by different types of studies needed to progress development through the lifecycle of the product is given in Section 4. In Section 5, important elements of clinical study design are described that reflect the variety of designs used in drug development as well as the range of data sources available. Section 6 addresses study conduct, ensuring the safety of study participants, and study reporting. Some considerations for identifying factors that are critical to the quality of a study are provided in Section 7.

The ICH Efficacy guidelines are an integrated set of guidance covering the planning, design, conduct, safety, analysis, and reporting of clinical studies. ICH E8 provides an overall introduction to clinical development, designing quality into clinical studies and focusing on those factors critical to the quality of the studies. The guidelines should be considered and used in an integrated, holistic way rather than focusing on only one guideline or subsection.

For the purposes of this document, a clinical study is meant to refer to a study of one or more medicinal products in humans, conducted at any point in a product's lifecycle, both prior to and following marketing authorisation. The focus is on clinical studies to support regulatory decisions, recognizing these studies may also inform health policy decisions, clinical practice guidelines, or other actions. The term "drug" should be considered synonymous with therapeutic, preventative, or diagnostic medicinal products. The term "drug approval" refers to obtaining marketing authorisation for the drug.

2. GENERAL PRINCIPLES

2.1 Protection of Clinical Study Participants

Important principles of ethical conduct of clinical studies and the protection of participants, including special populations, have their origins in the Declaration of Helsinki and should be observed in the conduct of all human clinical investigations. These principles are stated in other ICH guidelines, in particular, ICH E6-Good Clinical Practice.

As further described in the E6 guideline, the investigator and sponsor have responsibilities for the protection of study participants together with the Institutional Review Board/Independent Ethics Committee.

The confidentiality of information that could identify participants should be protected in accordance with the applicable regulatory and legal requirement(s).

Before initiating a clinical study, sufficient information should be available to ensure that the drug is acceptably safe for the planned study in humans. Emerging non-clinical, clinical, and pharmaceutical quality data should be reviewed and evaluated, as they become available, by qualified experts to assess the potential implications for the safety of study participants. Ongoing and future studies should be appropriately adjusted as needed, to take new knowledge into consideration and to protect study participants. Throughout drug development, care should be taken to ensure all study procedures and assessments are necessary from a scientific viewpoint and do not place undue burden on study participants.

2.2 Scientific Approach in Clinical Study Design, Planning, Conduct, Analysis, and Reporting

The essence of clinical research is to ask important questions and answer them with appropriate studies. The primary objectives of any study should reflect the research questions and be clear and explicitly stated. Clinical studies should be designed, planned, conducted, analysed, and reported according to sound scientific principles to achieve their objectives.

Quality of a clinical study is considered in this document as fitness for purpose. The purpose of a clinical study is to generate reliable information to answer the research questions and support decision making while protecting study participants. The quality of the information generated should therefore be sufficient to support good decision making.

Quality by design in clinical research sets out to ensure that the quality of a study is driven proactively by designing quality into the study protocol and processes. This involves the use of a prospective, multidisciplinary approach to promote the quality of protocol and process design in a manner proportionate to the risks involved, and clear communication of how this will be achieved.

Across the product lifecycle, different types of studies will be conducted with different objectives and designs and may involve different data sources. For purposes of this guideline, development planning is considered to cover the entire product lifecycle (Section 4). The Annex provides a broad categorisation of study type by objective within the different stages of drug development. Studies should be rigorously designed to address the study objectives with careful attention to the design elements, such as the choice of study population and response variables and the use of methods to minimize biases in the findings (Section 5).

The cardinal logic behind serially conducted studies is that the results of prior studies should inform the plan of later studies. Emerging data will frequently prompt a modification of the development strategy. For example, results of a confirmatory study may suggest a need for additional human pharmacology studies.

The availability of multi-regional data as a result of the increased globalisation of drug development programmes, facilitated by the harmonisation of ICH Guidelines, minimises the need to conduct individual studies in different regions. The results of a study are often used in regulatory submissions in multiple regions, and the design should also consider the relevance of the study results for regions other than the one(s) in which the study is conducted. Further guidance is provided by ICH E5 Ethnic Factors, ICH E6, and ICH E17 Multi-Regional Clinical Trials.

Early engagement with regulatory authorities to understand local/ regional requirements and expectations is encouraged and will facilitate the ability to design quality into the study.

2.3   Patient Input into Drug Development

Consulting with patients and/or patient organisations during drug development can help to ensure that patients' perspectives are captured. The views of patients (or of their caregivers/parents) can be valuable throughout all phases of drug development. Involving patients early in the design of a study is likely to increase trust in the study, facilitate recruitment, and promote adherence. Patients also provide their perspective of living with a condition, which may contribute to the determination, for example, of endpoints that are meaningful to patients, selection of the appropriate population and duration of the study, and use of acceptable comparators. This ultimately supports the development of drugs that are better tailored to patients' needs.

3. DESIGNING QUALITY INTO CLINICAL STUDIES

The quality by design approach to clinical research (Section 3.1) involves focusing on critical to quality factors to ensure the protection of the rights, safety, and wellbeing of study participants, the generation of reliable and meaningful results, and the management of risks to those factors using a risk-proportionate approach (Section 3.2). The approach is supported by the establishment of an appropriate framework for the identification and review of critical to quality factors (Section 3.3) at the time of design and planning of the study, and throughout its conduct, analysis, and reporting.

3.1 Quality by Design of Clinical Studies

Quality is a primary consideration in the design, planning, conduct, analysis, and reporting of clinical studies and a necessary component of clinical development programmes. The likelihood that a clinical study will answer the research questions while preventing important errors can be dramatically improved through prospective attention to the design of all components of the study protocol, procedures, associated operational plans and training. Activities such as document and data review and monitoring, where conducted retrospectively, are an important part of a quality assurance process; but, even when combined with audits, they are not sufficient to ensure quality of a clinical study.

Good planning and implementation of a clinical study also derive from attention to the design elements of clinical studies as described in Section 5, such as:

- the need for clear pre-defined study objectives that address the primary scientific question(s);

- selection of appropriate participants that have the disease, condition, or molecular/genetic profile that is being studied;
- use of approaches to minimise bias, such as randomization, blinding or masking, and/or control of confounding;
- endpoints that are well-defined, measurable, clinically meaningful, and relevant to patients.

Operational criteria are also important, such as ensuring a clear understanding of the feasibility of the study, selection of suitable investigator sites, quality of specialised analytical and testing facilities and procedures, and processes that ensure data integrity.

3.2   Critical to Quality Factors

A basic set of factors relevant to ensuring study quality should be identified for each study. Emphasis should be given to those factors that stand out as critical to study quality. These critical to quality factors are attributes of a study whose integrity is fundamental to the protection of study participants, the reliability and interpretability of the study results, and the decisions made based on the study results. These quality factors are considered to be critical because, if their integrity were to be undermined by errors of design or conduct, the reliability or ethics of decision-making based on the results of the study would also be undermined. Critical to quality factors should also be considered holistically, so that dependencies among them can be identified. Section 7 of this document provides considerations that can help identify critical to quality factors for a study.

The design of a clinical study should reflect the state of knowledge and experience with the drug; the condition to be treated, diagnosed or prevented; the underlying biological mechanism (of both the condition and the treatment); and the population for which the drug is intended. As research progresses, knowledge increases and uncertainties about the pharmacology, safety and efficacy of a drug decrease. Knowledge of the drug at any point in development will continually inform the identification of critical to quality factors and control processes used to manage them.

The sponsor and other parties designing quality into a clinical study should identify the critical to quality factors. Having identified those factors, it is important to determine the risks that threaten their integrity and decide whether they can be accepted or should be mitigated, based on their probability, detectability and impact. Where it is decided that risks should be mitigated, the necessary control processes should be put in place and communicated, and the necessary actions taken to mitigate the risks. The term risk is used here in the context of general risk management methodology applicable to all factors of a study.

Proactive communication of the critical to quality factors and risk mitigation activities will support understanding of priorities and resource allocation by the sponsor and investigator sites. Proactive support (e.g., training to site staff, relevant to their role, and description of critical to quality factors and potential mitigation measures in the protocol) will enhance correct implementation of study protocol, procedures, and associated operational plans and process design.

Perfection in every aspect of an activity is rarely achievable or can only be achieved by use of resources that are out of proportion to the benefit obtained. The quality factors should be prioritised to identify those that are critical to the study, at the time of the study design, and study procedures should be proportionate to the risks inherent in the study and the importance of the information collected. The critical to quality factors should be clear and should not be cluttered with minor issues (e.g., due to extensive secondary objectives or processes/data collection not linked to the proper protection of the study participants and/or primary study objectives).

3.3 Approach to Identifying the Critical to Quality Factors

A key aspect of a quality approach to study design is to ask whether the objectives being addressed by the study are clearly articulated; whether the study is designed to meet the research question it sets out to address; whether these questions are meaningful to patients; and whether the study hypotheses are specific and scientifically valid. The approach to the identification of the critical to quality factors should consider whether those objectives can be met, well and most efficiently, by the chosen design and data sources. Patient consultation early in the study design process can contribute to this approach and ultimately help to identify the critical to quality factors. Study designs should be operationally feasible and avoid unnecessary complexity. Protocols and case report forms/data collection methods should enable the study to be conducted as designed and avoid unnecessary data collection.

Identification of critical to quality factors will be enhanced by approaches that include the following elements:

3.3.1 Establishing a Culture that Supports Open Dialogue

Creating a culture that values and rewards critical thinking and open, proactive dialogue about what is critical to quality for a particular study or development programme, going beyond sole reliance on tools and checklists, is encouraged. Open dialogue can facilitate the development of innovative methods for ensuring quality.

Inflexible, "one size fits all" approaches should be discouraged. Standardised operating procedures are necessary and beneficial for conducting good quality clinical studies, but study specific strategies and actions are also needed to effectively and efficiently support quality in a study.

Evidence used to inform the study design should be gathered and reviewed, before and during the study, in a transparent manner, while acknowledging gaps in data and conflicting data, where present and known, and anticipating the possible emergence of such gaps or conflicts.

3.3.2 Focusing on Activities Essential to the Study

Efforts should be focused on activities that are essential to the reliability and meaningfulness of study outcomes for patients and public health, and the safe, ethical conduct of the study for participants. Consideration should be given to eliminating nonessential activities and data collection from the study to increase quality by simplifying conduct, improving study efficiency, and targeting resources to critical areas. Resources should be deployed to identify and prevent or control errors that matter.

3.3.3 Engaging Stakeholders in Study Design

Clinical study design is best informed by input from a broad range of stakeholders, including patients and healthcare providers. It should be open to challenge by subject matter experts and stakeholders from outside, as well as within, the sponsor organisation.

The process of building quality into the study may be informed by participation of those directly involved in successful completion of the study such as clinical investigators, study coordinators and other site staff, and patients/patient organisations. Clinical investigators and potential study participants have valuable insights into the feasibility of enrolling participants who meet proposed eligibility criteria, whether scheduled study visits and procedures may be overly burdensome and lead to early dropouts, and the general relevance of study endpoints and study settings to the targeted patient population. They may also provide insight into the value of a treatment in the context of ethical issues, culture, region, demographics, and other characteristics of subgroups within a targeted patient population.

Early engagement with regulatory authorities is encouraged, particularly when a study has novel elements considered critical to quality (e.g., defining patient populations, procedures, or endpoints).

3.3.4 Reviewing Critical to Quality Factors

Accumulated experience and knowledge, together with periodic review of critical to quality factors should be used to determine whether adjustments to risk control mechanisms are needed, because new or unanticipated issues may arise once the study has begun.

Studies with adaptive features and/or interim decision points need specific attention during proactive planning and ongoing review of critical to quality factors, and risk management (ICH E9 Statistical Principles for Clinical Trials).

3.3.5 Critical to Quality Factors in Operational Practice

The foundation of a successful study is a protocol that is both scientifically sound and operationally feasible. A feasibility assessment involves consideration of study design and implementation elements that could impact the successful completion of clinical development from an operational perspective.

Feasibility considerations also include but are not limited to regional differences in medical practice and patient populations, the availability of qualified investigators/site personnel with experience in conducting a clinical study (ICH E6), availability of equipment and facilities required to successfully conduct the study, availability of the targeted patient population, and ability to enrol a sufficient number of participants to meet the study objectives. The retention and follow up of study participants are also key critical to quality factors. Consideration of these and other critical to quality factors relating to study feasibility can inform study design and enhance quality implementation.

4. DRUG DEVELOPMENT PLANNING

This section provides general principles to consider in drug development planning. Drug development planning adheres to the principles of scientific research and good study design that ensure the reliability and interpretability of results. Efficient drug development includes appropriately planned interactions with regulatory authorities throughout development to ensure alignment with requirements for product quality and to support approval in the condition or disease, including possible post-approval studies to address remaining questions. Throughout this process there is critical attention to the protection of the rights, safety and wellbeing of study participants.

Drug development planning builds on knowledge acquired throughout the investigational process to reduce levels of uncertainty as the process moves from target identification through non-clinical and clinical evaluation. Such planning encompasses quality of medicinal product, including chemistry, manufacturing and controls (CMC), and non-clinical and clinical studies (pre and post-approval). Modelling and simulation may inform drug development throughout the process. Planning may also include regional considerations for product introduction into the market, such as health technology assessments.

It is important to ensure that the experiences, perspectives, needs, and priorities of relevant stakeholders relating to the development and evaluation of the drug throughout its lifecycle are captured and meaningfully incorporated into drug development planning.

Clinical development may also feature requirements for co-development of validated biomarkers, diagnostic testing, or devices that facilitate the safe and effective use of a drug.

The types of studies that may contribute to drug development are described in subsections 4.2 and 4.3 and summarised in the Annex.

4.1 Quality of Investigational Medicinal Product

Ensuring adequate quality and characterisation of physicochemical properties of investigational medicinal product is an important element in planning a drug development programme and is addressed in ICH and regional quality guidelines. More extensive characterisation may be required for complex or biological products. Formulations should be well characterised in the drug development plan, including information on bioavailability, wherever feasible, and should be appropriate for the stage of drug development and the targeted patient population. Age-appropriate formulation development may be a consideration when clinical studies are planned in paediatric populations (ICH E11- E11A Clinical Trials in Pediatric Population).

Evaluation of the quality of a drug may extend to devices required for its administration or a companion diagnostic to identify the targeted population.

Changes in a product during development should be supported by comparability data to ensure the ability to interpret study results across the development programme. This includes establishing links between formulations through bioequivalence studies or other means.

4.2 Non-Clinical Studies

Guidance on non-clinical safety studies is provided in ICH M3 Nonclinical Safety Studies, ICH Safety (S) Guidelines and related Q&A

documents, as well as in regional guidance. The non- clinical assessment usually includes toxicology, carcinogenicity, immunogenicity, pharmacology, pharmacokinetics, and other evaluations to support clinical studies (and may encompass evidence generated in *in vivo* and *in vitro* models, and by modelling and simulation). The scope of non-clinical studies, and their timing with respect to clinical studies, depend on a variety of factors that inform further development, such as the drug's chemical or molecular properties; pharmacological basis of principal effects (mechanism of action); route(s) of administration; absorption, distribution, metabolism, and excretion (ADME); physiological effects on organ systems; dose/concentration-response relationships; metabolites; and duration of action and use. Use of the drug in special populations (e.g., pregnant or breast-feeding women, children) may require additional non-clinical assessments. Guidance for non-clinical safety studies to support human clinical studies in special populations should be reviewed (see, e.g., ICH S5 Reproductive Toxicology, S11 Nonclinical Paediatric Safety, and M3).

Assessment of the preclinical characteristics, including physiological and toxicological effects of the drug, serve to inform clinical study design and planned use in humans. Before proceeding to studies in humans there should be sufficient non-clinical information to support initial human doses and duration of exposure.

4.3   Clinical Studies

Clinical drug development, defined as studying the drug in humans, is conducted in a sequence that builds on knowledge accumulated from non-clinical and previous clinical studies. The structure of the drug development programme will be shaped by many considerations and comprised of studies with different objectives, different designs, and different dependencies. The Annex provides an illustrative list of example studies and their objectives. Although clinical drug development is often described as consisting of four temporal phases (phases 1- 4), it is important to appreciate that the phase concept is a description and not a requirement, and that the phases of drug development may overlap or be combined.

To develop new drugs efficiently, it is essential to identify their characteristics in the early stages of development and to plan an appropriate development programme based on this profile. Initial clinical studies may be more limited in size and duration to provide an early evaluation of short-term safety and tolerability as well as proof of concept of efficacy. These studies may provide pharmacodynamic, pharmacokinetic, and other information needed to choose a suitable dosage range and/or administration schedule to inform further clinical studies. As more information is known about the drug, clinical studies may expand in size and duration, may include more diverse study populations, and may include more secondary endpoints in addition to the primary measures of efficacy. Throughout development, new data may suggest the need for additional studies.

The use of biomarkers has the potential to facilitate the availability of safer and more effective drugs, to guide dose selection, and to enhance a drug's benefit-risk profile (see ICH E16 Qualification of Genomic Biomarkers) and may be considered throughout drug development. Clinical studies may evaluate the use of biomarkers to better target patients more likely to benefit and less likely to experience adverse reactions, or as intermediate endpoints that could predict clinical response.

The following subsections describe the types of studies that typically span clinical development from the first studies in humans through late development and post-approval.

4.3.1 Human Pharmacology

The protection of study participants should always be the first priority when designing early clinical studies, especially for the initial administration of an investigational product to humans (usually referred to as phase 1). These studies may be conducted in healthy volunteer participants or in a selected population of patients who have the condition or the disease, depending on drug properties and the objectives of the development programme.

These studies typically address one or a combination of the following aspects:

4.3.1.1 Estimation of Initial Safety and Tolerability

The initial and subsequent administration of a drug to humans is usually intended to determine the tolerability of the dose range expected to be evaluated in later clinical studies and to determine the nature of adverse reactions that can be expected. These studies typically include both single and multiple dose administration.

4.3.1.2 Pharmacokinetics

Characterisation of a drug's absorption, distribution, metabolism, and excretion continues throughout the development programme, but the preliminary characterisation is an essential early goal. Pharmacokinetic studies are particularly important to assess the clearance of the drug and to anticipate possible accumulation of parent drug or metabolites, interactions with metabolic enzymes and transporters, and potential drug-drug interactions. Some pharmacokinetic studies are commonly conducted in later phases to answer more specialised questions. For orally administered drugs, the study of food effects on bioavailability is important to inform the dosing instructions in relation to food. Obtaining pharmacokinetic information in sub-populations with potentially different metabolism or excretion, such as patients with renal or hepatic impairment, geriatric patients, children, and ethnic subgroups should be considered (ICH E4 Dose-Response Studies, E7 Clinical Trials in Geriatric Population, E11, and E5, respectively).

4.3.1.3 Pharmacodynamics & Early Measurement of Drug Activity

Depending on the drug and the endpoint of interest, pharmacodynamic studies and studies relating drug levels to response (PK/PD studies) may be conducted in healthy volunteer participants or in patients with the condition or disease. If there is an appropriate measure, pharmacodynamic data can provide early estimates of activity and efficacy and may guide the dosage and dose regimen in later studies.

4.3.2 *Exploratory and Confirmatory Safety and Efficacy Studies*

After initial clinical studies provide sufficient information on safety, clinical pharmacology and dose, exploratory and confirmatory studies (usually referred to as phases 2 and 3, respectively) are conducted to further evaluate both the safety and efficacy of the drug. Depending on the nature of the drug and the patient population, this objective may be combined in a single or small number of studies. Exploratory and confirmatory studies may use a variety of study designs depending on the objective of the study.

Exploratory studies are designed to investigate safety and efficacy in a selected population of patients for whom the drug is intended. Additionally, these studies aim to refine the effective dose(s) and regimen, refine the definition of the targeted population, provide a more robust safety profile for the drug, and include evaluation of potential study endpoints for subsequent studies. Exploratory studies may provide information on the identification and determination of factors that affect the treatment effect and, possibly combined with modelling and simulation, serve to support the design of later confirmatory studies.

Confirmatory studies are designed to confirm the preliminary evidence accumulated in earlier clinical studies that a drug is safe and effective for use for the intended indication and recipient population. These studies are often intended to provide an adequate basis for marketing approval, and to support adequate instructions for use of the drug and official product information. They aim to evaluate the drug in participants with or at risk of the condition or disease who represent those who will receive the drug once approved. This may include investigating subgroups of patients with frequently occurring or potentially relevant co- morbidities (e.g., cardiovascular disease, diabetes, hepatic and renal impairment) to characterise the safe and effective use of the drug in patients with these conditions.

Confirmatory studies may evaluate the efficacy and safety of more than one dose or the use of the drug in different stages of disease or in combination with one or more other drugs. If the intent is to administer a drug for a long period of time, then studies involving extended exposure to the drug should be conducted (ICH E1 Clinical Safety for Drugs used in Long-Term Treatment). Irrespective of the intended duration of administration, the duration of effect of the drug will also inform the duration of follow-up.

Study endpoints selected for confirmatory studies should be clinically relevant and reflect disease burden or be of adequate surrogacy for predicting disease burden or sequelae.

4.3.3 Special Populations

Some groups in the general population require additional investigation during drug development because they have unique risk/benefit considerations, or because they can be anticipated to need modification of the dose or schedule of a drug. ICH E5 and E17 provide a framework for evaluating the impact of ethnic factors on a drug's effect. Particular attention should be paid to the ethical considerations related to informed consent in vulnerable populations (ICH E6 and E11). Studies in special populations may be conducted during any phase of development to understand the drug effects in these populations. Some considerations of special populations are the following:

4.3.3.1 Investigations in pregnant women

Investigation of drugs that may be used in pregnancy is important. Where pregnant women volunteer to be enrolled in a clinical study, or a participant becomes pregnant while participating in a clinical study, follow-up evaluation of the pregnancy and its outcome and the reporting of outcomes are necessary.

4.3.3.2 Investigations in lactating women

Excretion of the drug or its metabolites into human milk should be examined where applicable and feasible. When nursing mothers are enrolled in clinical studies their babies are usually also monitored for the effects of the drug.

4.3.3.3 Investigations in children

ICH E11 provides an outline of critical issues in paediatric drug development and approaches to the safe, efficient, and ethical study of drugs in paediatric populations.

4.3.3.4 Investigations in geriatric populations

ICH E7 provides an outline of critical issues in developing drugs for use in geriatric populations and approaches to their safe, efficient, and ethical study.

4.3.4 Post-Approval Studies

After the approval of a drug, additional studies may be conducted to further understand the safety and efficacy of the drug in its approved indication (usually referred to as phase 4). These are studies that were not considered necessary for approval but are often important for optimising the drug's use. They may be of any type but should have valid scientific objectives. Post-approval studies may be conducted to address a regulatory requirement.

Post-approval studies may be performed to provide additional information on the efficacy, safety, and use of the drug in populations more diverse than included in the studies conducted prior to marketing authorisation. Studies with long-term follow-up or with comparisons to other treatment options or standards of care may provide important information on safety and efficacy. Commonly conducted studies include additional drug-drug interaction, dose-response or safety studies and studies designed to support use under the approved indication (e.g., mortality/morbidity studies, epidemiological studies). These studies may explore use of the drug in the real-world setting of clinical practice and may also inform health economics and health technology assessments.

4.4 Additional Development

After initial approval, drug development may continue with studies of new or modified indications in new patient populations, new dosage regimens, or new routes of administration. If a new dose, formulation, or combination is studied, additional non-clinical and/or human pharmacology studies may be indicated. Data from previous studies or from clinical experience with the approved drug may inform these programmes.

5. DESIGN ELEMENTS AND DATA SOURCES FOR CLINICAL STUDIES

Study objectives impact the choice of study design and data sources, which in turn impact the strength of a study to support regulatory decisions and clinical practice. As discussed in Section 4, there are a wide variety of study objectives in drug development. Similarly, there is a wide range of study designs and data sources to address these objectives. Sections 5.1 through 5.6 discuss key elements that may be used to define the study design, and Section 5.7 discusses the various data sources that may be used for the study.

Clear objectives will help to specify the study design, and conversely, the process of specifying the design may help to further clarify the objectives. At the design stage, the objectives may need to be modified if substantial practical considerations and limitations or other risks to critical to quality factors are identified. The study objectives are further refined through specification of estimands. Estimands, discussed in ICH E9(R1) Addendum: Statistical Principles for Clinical Trials, provide a precise description of the treatment effects reflecting the clinical questions posed by the study objectives. The estimand summarises at a population level what the outcomes would be in the same patients under the different treatment conditions being compared.

An important distinction between studies is whether the allocation of individuals to the study drug(s) is controlled by the study procedures or allocation to the drug is not controlled but exposure to the drug(s) is observed in the study. In this document, the former case is referred to as an interventional study and the latter case is referred to as an observational study.

Interventional studies, and in particular randomised studies, play a central role in drug development, as they can better control biases. The designs of randomised studies range from simple parallel group designs to more complex variants. For example, adaptive design studies allow prospectively planned modifications to the study, such as changes in the population studied or changes in doses of the drug studied over the course of the study, based on accumulating data. Master protocol studies allow for the investigation of multiple drugs or multiple conditions under a shared framework. Platform studies allow for multiple drugs to be investigated in a continuous manner, with different drugs entering the study at different times and leaving the study based on pre-specified decision rules.

Studies without randomisation (whether interventional or observational) can play a role as well in certain settings when randomisation is not feasible. Observational studies are often conducted post-approval but can be of utility as complementary sources of evidence during development and across the life cycle of a drug.

Along with the breadth of study designs, there are multiple sources of data that studies may employ. Traditionally, studies have used study-specific data collection processes. Data such as that obtained from electronic medical records or digital health technologies may be leveraged to increase the efficiency of studies or generalisability of study results.

This section presents important elements that define the design of a clinical study including population, treatment, control group, response variable, methods to reduce bias, statistical analysis, and data sources. It is intended to assist in identifying the critical to quality factors necessary to achieve the study objectives, while also enabling flexibility in study design and promoting efficiency in study conduct. Although the focus is on interventional studies, the discussion is intended to apply to both interventional and observational studies. The elements outlined here are expected to be relevant to study types and data sources that are used in clinical studies now and that may be developed in the future.

5.1 Study Population

The population to be studied should be chosen to support the study objectives and is defined through the inclusion and exclusion criteria for the study. The degree to which a study succeeds in enrolling the desired population will impact the ability of the study to meet its objectives.

The study population may be narrowly defined to reduce the risk to study participants or to maximise the sensitivity of the study for detecting a certain effect. Conversely, it may be broadly defined to more closely represent the diverse populations for which the drug is intended. In general, studies conducted early in a development programme, when little is known about the safety of the drug, are more homogeneous in study population definitions. Studies conducted in the later phases of drug development or post-approval are often more heterogeneous in study population definitions. Such studies should involve participants who are representative of the diverse populations which will receive the intervention in clinical practice. Available knowledge about participant characteristics that may predict disease outcomes or effects of the intervention can be used to further define the study population.

The number of participants (sample size) in a study should be large enough to provide a reliable answer to the questions addressed (see ICH E9). This number is usually determined by the primary objective of the study. If the sample size is determined on some other basis, then this should be made clear and justified. For example, a sample size determined to address safety questions or meet important secondary objectives may need larger numbers of participants than needed for addressing the primary efficacy question (see ICH E1). If study objectives include obtaining information on certain subgroups, then efforts should be made to ensure adequate representation of these subgroups.

5.2 Treatment Description

The treatment(s), including controls, under study should be described explicitly and specifically. These might be individual treatments (including different doses or regimens), combinations of treatments, or no treatments, and can include specification of background treatments. The definition of treatments should align with the objectives of the study (ICH E9(R1)). For example, if the objective of the study is to understand the effect of the treatment in clinical practice, the study may specify that the background treatment, if any, is up to the discretion of the participants and healthcare providers. If the objectives are to understand the effect of the drug when added to a specific background treatment, the background treatment should be defined explicitly and specifically for all groups including controls.

5.3   Choice of Control Group

The major purpose of a control group is to separate the effect of the treatment(s) from the effects of other factors such as natural course of the disease, other medical care received, or observer or patient expectations (E10 Choice of Control Group in Clinical Trials). The treatment effect of interest may be the effect relative to not receiving the drug or the effect relative to receiving other therapies. Comparisons may be made with placebo, no treatment, standard of care, other treatments, or different doses of the drug under investigation.

The source of control group data may be internal or external to the study. The intent of using an internal control group is to help ensure that the only differences between treatment groups are due to the treatment they receive and not due to differences in the selection of participants, the timing and measurement of study outcomes, or other differences. A special case of an internal control group is when each participant serves as their own internal control by receiving the drug and control at different points of time. With use of an external control group, individuals are selected from an external source, and the individuals may have been treated at an earlier time (historical control group) or during the same time but in another setting than participants in the study.

Important limitations of the use of external controls are discussed in ICH E10. Particular care is needed to minimise the likelihood of erroneous inference. The use of an external control requires that the disease course is well known and predictable. External control individuals may differ from study participants with respect to demographic and background characteristics (e.g., medical history, concurrent diseases). In addition, external control individuals may differ from participants in the study with respect to concurrent care and the measurement of study outcomes and other data elements. Because the use of internal controls generally mitigates the potential for bias better than external controls, particularly in conjunction with randomisation, the suitability of the use and choice of external control should be carefully considered and justified. Section 5.5 discusses the sources of bias which can arise in observational studies and is relevant to the use of external controls.

Participant level data may not be available for some choices of external control groups. Summary measures may be available to form the basis of comparisons with treated participants to estimate drug effects and test hypotheses about those effects. There is, however, less ability to control for differences in characteristics between study individuals in the external control group and study participants in the internal treatment groups in making these comparisons or examining the quality and completeness of individual data elements. Additionally, there may not be the ability to examine subgroups or modify the response variable to be consistent with the response variable used in the study.

5.4   Response Variables

A response variable is an attribute of interest that may be affected by the drug. The response variable may relate to pharmacokinetics, pharmacodynamics, efficacy, or safety of the drug, or to the use of the drug including, for example, in adherence to risk minimisation measures post- approval. Study endpoints are the response variables that are chosen to assess drug effects.

The primary endpoint should be capable of providing clinically relevant and convincing evidence related to the primary objective of the study (ICH E9). Secondary endpoints are either supportive measurements related to the primary objective or measurements of effects related to the secondary objectives. Exploratory endpoints are used to further explain or to support study findings or to explore new hypotheses for later research. The choice of endpoints should be meaningful for the intended population and may also take into account the views of patients. The definition of each study endpoint should be specific and include how and at what time points in a participant's treatment course of the drug and follow-up it is ascertained.

Knowledge of the drug, along with the clinical context and purpose of a given study affect what response variables should be collected. For example, a proof-of-concept study of relatively short duration may employ a pharmacodynamic outcome rather than the outcome of primary interest (ICH E9). A larger study of longer duration could then be used to confirm a clinically meaningful effect on the outcome of primary interest. In other cases, such as a study where the safety profile of the drug is well characterised, the extent of safety data collection may be tailored to the objectives of the study.

5.5 Methods to Reduce Bias

The study design should address potential sources of bias that can undermine the reliability of results. Although different types of studies are subject to different sources of bias, this section addresses some common sources. ICH E9 discusses principles for controlling and reducing bias mainly in the context of interventional studies.

In studies with internal control groups, randomisation is used to ensure comparability of treatment groups, thereby minimising the possibility of bias in treatment assignment.

Randomisation at the start of the study addresses differences between the groups at the time of randomisation but does not prevent bias due to differences arising during the study. Events after randomisation (particularly intercurrent events (ICH E9(R1)) may affect the validity and interpretation of comparisons between treatment groups. Examples include treatment discontinuation or use of rescue medications. There may also be differences in the follow-up patterns between the groups due to participants in one group discontinuing the study at different rates, because of, for example, adverse events or perceived lack of efficacy. Careful consideration of the potential for intercurrent events to occur during the study and their impact will help with the identification of critical to quality factors, such as reducing study discontinuation, continuing data collection following treatment discontinuation, and retrieving data after study discontinuation, if appropriate. It is important when defining the treatment effect (estimand) to account for the occurrence of intercurrent events.

Concealing the treatment assignments (blinding) limits the occurrence of conscious or unconscious bias in the conduct and interpretation of a clinical study that may affect the course of treatment, monitoring, endpoint ascertainment, and participants' responses. In a single-blind study the investigator is aware of the treatment, but the participant is not. When the investigators who are involved in the treatment or clinical evaluation of the participants are also unaware of the treatment assignments, the study is referred to as double-blind. In an open- label study, the consequences of the lack of blinding may be reduced through the use of pre- specified decision rules for aspects of study conduct, such as recruitment, treatment assignment, participant management, safety reporting, and response variable ascertainment. Blinding for staff at the study sites or sponsor should be implemented where feasible.

Knowledge of interim results (whether individual or treatment group level) has the potential to introduce bias or influence the conduct of the study and interpretation of study results. Specific considerations related to information flow and confidentiality are therefore necessary.

Observational studies introduce unique challenges to the assessment and control of bias. These include ensuring that the individuals have the condition under study and ensuring comparability between treatment groups, in prognostic factors associated with the choice of therapies, in the ascertainment of response variables, and in post-baseline concomitant patient care. These challenges may also exist with the use of external controls in an interventional study. Methods exist that may mitigate some of these challenges and should be considered during the design phase.

5.6   Statistical Analysis

The statistical analysis of a study encompasses important elements necessary to achieving the study objectives. The specification and documentation of the statistical analysis are important for ensuring the integrity of the study findings. The principal features of the statistical analysis should be planned during the design of the study and should be clearly specified in a protocol written before the study begins (ICH E9). Full details of the planned statistical analysis should be specified and documented before knowledge of the study results that may reveal the drug effects, which may be accomplished using a separate statistical analysis plan. The protocol should define the estimand(s) following the framework established in ICH E9(R1).

Statistical analyses of primary and secondary endpoints that address key study objectives with respect to both efficacy and safety should be described in the protocol, including any interim analyses and/or planned design adaptations. Other statistical aspects of the study that should be described in the protocol include the analytical methods for any planned estimation and tests of hypotheses about the drug effect and a justification of the sample size.

The statistical analysis should include pre-specified sensitivity analyses for assessing the impact of the assumptions made for the primary and important secondary analyses on the results of the study (E9(R1)). For example, if the analysis relies on a particular assumption about the reasons for missing data, sensitivity analyses should be planned to assess the impact of that assumption on the study results. In the case of observational studies, sensitivity analyses might, for example, consider additional potential confounders.

For double-blind studies, the statistical analysis plan should be finalised before treatment assignments are revealed. Therefore, if a study includes one or more interim analyses, the planned statistical analysis should not be changed after an interim analysis that involves unblinding. For open-label and single-blind studies, details pertaining to the primary and important secondary analyses would ideally be finalised before the first participant is randomised or allocated to study intervention.

Pre-specification of the analysis approach is particularly important for studies that make use of existing data sources rather than primary data collection (Section 5.7), not only for the statistical analysis planned for the study but also for any feasibility analysis to assess the applicability of the existing data. For example, for a single-arm interventional study with an external control, the specifics of the external control should be defined prior to the conduct of the interventional aspect of the study. Pre-specification of the analysis should be in place so that any review of the existing data sources prior to the design of the study does not threaten the study integrity.

The statistical analysis should be carried out in accordance with the prospectively defined analysis plan, and all deviations from the plan should be indicated in the study report (E3 Clinical Study Reports).

5.7   Study Data

Study data comprise all information generated, collected, or used in the context of the study ranging from existing source data to study-specific assessments. The study data should contain the necessary information to conduct the statistical analysis specified in the protocol and statistical analysis plan, as well as to monitor for participant safety, protocol adherence, and data integrity.

Study data can be broadly classified into two types: (1) data generated specifically for the present study (primary data collection) and (2) data obtained from sources external to the present study (secondary data use). Data generated for the study may be collected via case report forms, laboratory measurements, electronic patient reported outcomes, or mobile health tools. Examples of external sources of data include historical clinical studies, national death databases, disease and drug registries, claims data, and medical and administrative records from routine medical practice. A study may make use of both types of data.

For all data sources, procedures to ensure the protection of personal data of the individuals being studied should be implemented. The study protocol, and if applicable the informed consent, should explicitly address the protection of personal data. Regulations related to protection of individuals' data need to be followed. When considering data from external sources, it is important to ascertain whether the regulatory authorities accept the use of such data for purposes other than the original intent.

Study data should be of sufficient quality to address the objectives of the study and, in interventional studies, to monitor participant safety. Data quality attributes include consistency (uniformity of ascertainment over time), accuracy (correctness of collection, transmission, and processing), and completeness (lack of missing information). These aspects should be proactively considered during study planning by identifying the factors, critical to the quality of the study, associated with data sourcing, collection, and processing.

The use of standards for data recording and coding (or recoding) is important to support data reliability, facilitate correct analysis and interpretation of results, and promote data sharing. Internationally accepted data standards exist for many sources of study data and should be used where applicable.

With primary data collection, the methods and standards established for use at the point of capture and the subsequent processing provide an opportunity to prospectively ensure the quality of the data.

With secondary data use, the relevance of the available data should be considered and clearly described in the study protocol. For example, when using existing electronic health record data to ascertain the study endpoint rather than through primary data collection, information in the health record about outcomes may need to be converted to the study endpoint.

In some cases, secondary data use may not be sufficient for all aspects of the study and may need to be supplemented by primary data collection. The quality of data collected for a different purpose should be evaluated when re-used in the context of the present study. Careful quality control processes may have been applied during their acquisition; where used, those processes were not necessarily designed with the objectives of the present study in mind.

There are several additional considerations with secondary data use. For example, methods to conceal the treatment should be considered when selecting and prior to analysing data from external sources. As another example, absence of affirmative information on a condition or event does not necessarily mean the condition or event is not present. There may also be a delay between the occurrence of events and their appearance in existing data sources. To the extent possible, uncertainties and potential sources of bias should be addressed at the study design stage, during data analysis, and in the interpretation of the study results.

6. CONDUCT, SAFETY MONITORING, AND REPORTING

6.1 Study Conduct

The principles and approaches set out in this guideline, including those of quality by design, should inform the approach taken to the conduct and reporting of clinical studies. Risk proportionate mitigation measures should be employed to ensure the integrity of the critical to quality factors.

6.1.1 Protocol Adherence

Adherence to the study protocol and other relevant documents is essential, and many aspects of adherence should be considered among the study's critical to quality factors. Successful application of the quality by design principles may minimise the need for modifications to the protocol and make adherence throughout the study more likely. If modification of the protocol becomes necessary, a clear description of the rationale for the modification should be provided in a protocol amendment, and the impact of the modification on study conduct should be carefully considered.

6.1.2 Training

Individuals involved in study conduct should receive training commensurate with their role in the study and this training should occur prior to their becoming involved in the study. Updated training or retraining may be needed to address issues related to critical to quality factors observed during the course of the study, and/or implement protocol modifications.

6.1.3 Data Management

The manner and timelines in which study data are collected and managed are critical contributors to overall study data quality. Operational checks, centralised data monitoring, and statistical surveillance can identify important data quality issues for corrective action. Data management procedures should account for the diversity of data sources in use for clinical studies (Section 5.7). For interventional clinical studies, further guidance on data management is available in ICH E6.

6.1.4 Access to Interim Data

Inappropriate access to data during the conduct of the study may compromise study integrity (Sections 5.5 and 5.6 and ICH E9). In studies with planned interim analyses, special attention should be given to which individuals have access to the data and results. Even in studies without planned interim analyses, special attention should be paid to any ongoing monitoring of unblinded data to avoid inappropriate access.

6.2 Participant Safety during Study Conduct

Important standards of ethical conduct and the protection of participants in clinical studies are described in Section 2.1. This section describes safety related considerations during the conduct of the study.

6.2.1 Safety Monitoring

The goals of safety monitoring are to protect study participants and to characterise the safety profile of the drug. Procedures and systems for the identification, monitoring, and reporting of safety concerns during the study should be clearly specified. The approach should reflect the type and objectives of the study, the risks to the study participants and what is known about the drug and the study population. Guidance is available on reporting of safety data to appropriate authorities and on the content and timing of safety reports (ICH E2-E2F Pharmacovigilance, and, for interventional clinical trials in particular, ICH E6).

6.2.2   Withdrawal Criteria

Clear criteria for stopping treatment or study procedures for a study participant while remaining in the study are necessary to ensure the protection of the participants but should also minimise loss of critical data.

6.2.3   Data Monitoring Committee

An important component of safety monitoring in many clinical studies is the use of an independent data monitoring committee. This group monitors accumulating data while the study is being conducted to make recommendations on whether to continue, modify, or terminate a study.

During programme planning, the need for an independent data monitoring committee to monitor safety data across studies in a development programme should also be assessed. If a data monitoring committee is needed for either an individual study or across the development programme, procedures governing its operation and, in particular the review of unblinded data in an interventional trial, while preserving study integrity (ICH E9) should be established prior to study start.

6.3   Study Reporting

Clinical studies and their results should be adequately reported using formats appropriate for the type of study (interventional or observational studies) and information being reported. ICH E3 focuses particularly on the report format for interventional clinical trials, but the basic principles may be applied to other types of clinical studies (ICH E3 Q&A). The design of the study report should be part of the quality by design process. The report should describe the critical to quality factors in the study. The reporting of study results should be comprehensive, accurate, and timely.

Consideration should be given to providing a factual summary of the overall study results to study participants in an objective, balanced and nonpromotional manner, including relevant safety information and any limitations of the study. In addition, consideration could be given to providing individual participants with information about their study specific results (e.g., their treatment arm, test results). The information should be conveyed by someone involved in the health management of the participant (e.g., the clinical investigator). Participants should be informed about the information they will receive and when they will receive it at the time of providing informed consent.

The transparency of clinical research in drug development includes the registration of clinical studies, before they start, on publicly accessible and recognised databases, and the public posting of clinical study results. Adopting such practices for observational studies also promotes transparency. Making objective and unbiased information publicly available can benefit public health in general, as well as the indicated patient populations, through enhancing clinical research, reducing unnecessary clinical studies, and informing decisions in clinical practice.

7. CONSIDERATIONS IN IDENTIFYING CRITICAL TO QUALITY FACTORS

The identification of critical to quality factors should be supported by proactive, cross- functional discussions and decision making at the time of study planning, as described in Section 3. Different factors will stand out as critical for different types of studies, following the concepts introduced in Sections 4 through 6.

In designing a study, the following aspects should be considered, where applicable, to support the identification of critical to quality factors:

- Engagement of all relevant stakeholders, including patients, is considered during study planning and design.
- The prerequisite non-clinical studies, and where applicable, clinical studies, are complete and adequate to support the study being designed.
- The study objectives address relevant scientific questions appropriate for a given study's role in the development

programme, taking into account the accumulated knowledge about the product.

- The clinical study design supports a meaningful comparison of the effects of the drug when compared to the chosen control group.
- Adequate measures are used to protect participants' rights, safety, and welfare (informed consent process, Institutional Review Board/Ethics Committee review, investigator and clinical study site training, pseudonymisation).
- Information provided to the study participants should be clear and understandable.
- Competencies and training required for the study by sponsor and investigator staff, relevant to their role, should be identified.
- The feasibility of the study should be assessed to ensure the study is operationally viable.
- The number of participants included, the duration of the study, and the frequency of study visits are sufficient to support the study objective.
- The eligibility criteria should be reflective of the study objectives and be well documented in the clinical study protocol.
- The protocol specifies the collection of data needed to meet the study objectives, understand the benefit/risk of the drug, and monitor participant safety.
- The choice of response variables and the methods to assess them are well-defined and support evaluation of the effects of the drug.
- Clinical study procedures include adequate measures to minimize bias (e.g., randomization, blinding).
- The statistical analysis plan is pre-specified and defines the analysis methods appropriate for the endpoints and the populations of interest.
- Systems and processes are in place that support the study conduct to ensure the integrity of critical study data.
- The extent and nature of study monitoring are tailored to the specific study design and objectives and the need to ensure participants' safety.

- The need for and appropriate role of a data monitoring committee is assessed.
- The reporting of the study results is planned, comprehensive, accurate, timely, and publicly accessible.

These considerations are not exhaustive and may not apply to all studies. Other aspects may need to be considered to identify the critical to quality factors for each individual study.

ANNEX: TYPES OF CLINICAL STUDIES

Drug development is ideally a logical, stepwise process in which information from early studies is used to support and plan later studies. The actual sequence of studies conducted in a particular drug development programme, however, may reflect different dependencies and overlapping study types. Studies may also involve adaptive designs (which may bridge or combine different study types as listed below) or designs that are intended to investigate multiple drugs or multiple indications or both (e.g., studies conducted under a master protocol). In the table below, types of clinical studies are categorised by objectives. Illustrative examples, not intended to be exhaustive or exclusive, are provided. Study objectives appearing under one type may also occur under another.

Type of Study	Objective(s) of Study	Study Examples
Human Pharmacology	• Assess tolerance and safety • Define/describe clinical PK[1] and PD[2] • Explore drug metabolism and drug interactions • Evaluate activity, assess immunogenicity • Assess renal/hepatic tolerance • Assess cardiac toxicity	• BA[3]/BE[4] studies under fasted/fed conditions • Dose-tolerance studies • Single and multiple-rising dose PK and/or PD studies • Drug-drug interaction studies • QTc prolongation study • Human factor studies for drug delivery devices
Exploratory	• Explore use for the intended indication • Estimate dose/dosing regimen for subsequent studies • Explore dose- response/ exposure-response relationship • Provide basis for confirmatory study design (e.g., targeted population, clinical endpoints, patient reported outcome measures, factors affecting treatment effects)	• Randomised controlled clinical trials of relatively short duration in well- defined narrow patient populations, using surrogate or pharmacological endpoints or clinical measures • Dose finding studies • Biomarker exploration studies • Studies to validate patient reported outcomes • Adaptive designs that may combine exploratory and confirmatory objectives

Confirmatory	• Demonstrate/confirm efficacy • Establish safety profile in larger, more representative patient populations • Provide an adequate basis for assessing the benefit/risk relationship to support licensing • Establish dose- response/exposure-response relationship • Establish safety profile and confirm efficacy in specific populations (e.g., paediatrics, elderly)	• Randomised controlled clinical trials to establish efficacy in larger, more representative patient populations • Dose-response studies • Clinical safety studies • Studies of mortality/morbidity outcomes • Studies in special populations • Studies that seek to demonstrate efficacy for multiple drugs in a single protocol
Post-Approval	• Extend understanding of benefit/risk relationship in general or special populations and/or environments • Identify less common adverse reactions • Refine dosing recommendations	• Comparative effectiveness studies • Long-term follow-up studies • Studies of mortality/morbidity or other additional endpoints • Large, simple randomised trials • Pharmacoeconomic studies • Pharmacoepidemiology studies • Observational studies of the use of the drug in clinical practice • Disease or drug registries
[1]PK - Pharmacokinetic [2]PD - Pharmacodynamic [3]BA studies - Bioavailability [4]BE studies - Bioequivalence		

ICH Guideline

Clinical Safety Data Management: Definitions and Standards for Expedited Reporting (E2A)

As published in the Federal Register
March 1, 1995

CONTENTS

KEY DATA ELEMENTS FOR INCLUSION IN EXPEDITED REPORTS OF SERIOUS ADVERSE DRUG REACTIONS

GUIDELINE FOR INDUSTRY[1]

CLINICAL SAFETY DATA MANAGEMENT: DEFINITIONS AND STANDARDS FOR EXPEDITED REPORTING[2]

I. *INTRODUCTION*

It is important to harmonize the way to gather and, if necessary, to take action on important clinical safety information arising during clinical development. Thus, agreed definitions and terminology, as well as procedures, will ensure uniform Good Clinical Practice standards in this area. The initiatives already undertaken for marketed medicines through the CIOMS-1 and CIOMS-2 Working Groups on expedited

---

[1] This guideline was developed within the Expert Working Group (Efficacy) of the International Conference on Harmonisation of Technical Requirements for Registration of Pharmaceuticals for Human Use (ICH) and has been subject to consultation by the regulatory parties, in accordance with the ICH process. This document has been endorsed by the ICH Steering Committee at Step 4 of the ICH process, October 27, 1994. At Step 4 of the process, the final draft is recommended for adoption to the regulatory bodies of the European Union, Japan and the USA. This guidance was published in the Federal Register on March 1, 1995 (60 FR 11284) and is applicable to both drug and biological products. In the past, guidelines have generally been issued under § 10.90(b) [21 CFR 10.90(b)], which provides for the use of guidelines to state the procedures or standards of general applicability that are not legal requirements but that are acceptable to FDA. The agency is now in the process of revising §10.90(b). Therefore, this guideline is not being issued under the authority of §10.90(b), and it does not create or confer any rights, privileges or benefits for or on any person, nor does it operate to bind FDA in any way. For additional copies of this guideline contact the Executive Secretariat Staff, HFD-8, Center for Drug Evaluation and Research, 7500 Standish Place, Rockville, MD 20855, 301-594-1012. An electronic version of this guideline is also available via Internet by connecting to the CDER FTP server (CDVS2.CDER.FDA.GOV) using the FTP protocol.
[2] The time frames and definitions in this guideline differ from those in the Code of Federal Regulations [21 CFR 314.80]. Until the regulations are revised, the time frames and definitions in the CFR should be followed.

(alert) reports and periodic safety update reporting, respectively, are important precedents and models. However, there are special circumstances involving medicinal products under development, especially in the early stages and before any marketing experience is available.

Conversely, it must be recognized that a medicinal product will be under various stages of development and/or marketing in different countries, and safety data from marketing experience will ordinarily be of interest to regulators in countries where the medicinal product is still under investigational only (Phase 1, 2, or 3) status. For this reason, it is both practical and well-advised to regard premarketing and post-marketing clinical safety reporting concepts and practices as interdependent, while recognizing that responsibility for clinical safety within regulatory bodies and companies may reside with different departments, depending on the status of the product (investigational vs. marketed).

There are two issues within the broad subject of clinical safety data management that are appropriate for harmonization at this time:

- the development of standard definitions and terminology for key aspects of clinical safety reporting, and
- the appropriate mechanism for handling expedited (rapid) reporting, in the investigational (i.e., pre-approval) phase.

The provisions of this guideline should be used in conjunction with other ICH Good Clinical Practice guidelines.

II. *DEFINITIONS AND TERMINOLOGY ASSOCIATED WITH CLINICAL SAFETY EXPERIENCE*

A. Basic Terms

Definitions for the terms adverse event (or experience), adverse reaction, and unexpected adverse reaction have previously been agreed to by consensus of the more than 30 Collaborating Centers of the WHO International Drug Monitoring Centre (Uppsala, Sweden). [Edwards, I.R., et al, "Harmonisation in Pharmacovigilance," Drug Safety 10(2): 93-102, 1994.] Although those definitions can pertain to situations involving clinical investigations, some minor modifications are necessary, especially to accommodate the pre-approval, development environment.

The following definitions, with input from the WHO Collaborative Centre, have been agreed:

1. Adverse Event (or Adverse Experience)
    Any untoward medical occurrence in a patient or clinical investigation subject administered a pharmaceutical product and which does not necessarily have to have a causal relationship with this treatment.

    An adverse event (AE) can therefore be any unfavorable and unintended sign (including an abnormal laboratory finding, for example), symptom, or disease temporally associated with the use of a medicinal product, whether or not considered related to the medicinal product.

2. Adverse Drug Reaction (ADR)
    In the pre-approval clinical experience with a new medicinal product or its new usages, particularly as the therapeutic dose(s) may not be established:

    all noxious and unintended responses to a medicinal product related to any dose should be considered adverse drug reactions.

The phrase "responses to a medicinal products" means that a causal relationship between a medicinal product and an adverse event is at least a reasonable possibility, i.e., the relationship cannot be ruled out.

Regarding marketed medicinal products, a well-accepted definition of an adverse drug reaction in the post-marketing setting is found in WHO Technical Report 498 [1972] and reads as follows:

> A response to a drug which is noxious and unintended and which occurs at doses normally used in man for prophylaxis, diagnosis, or therapy of disease or for modification of physiological function.

The old term "side effect" has been used in various ways in the past, usually to describe negative (unfavorable) effects, but also positive (favorable) effects. It is recommended that this term no longer be used and particularly should not be regarded as synonymous with adverse event or adverse reaction.

3. Unexpected Adverse Drug Reaction
    An adverse reaction, the nature or severity of which is not consistent with the applicable product information (e.g., Investigator's Brochure for an unapproved investigational medicinal product). See section III.C.

B. Serious Adverse Event or Adverse Drug Reaction

During clinical investigations, adverse events may occur which, if suspected to be medicinal product-related (adverse drug reactions), might be significant enough to lead to important changes in the way the medicinal product is developed (e.g., change in dose, population, needed monitoring, consent forms). This is particularly true for reactions which, in their most severe forms, threaten life or function. Such reactions should be reported promptly to regulators.

Therefore, special medical or administrative criteria are needed to define reactions that, either due to their nature ("serious") or due to the significant, unexpected information they provide, justify expedited reporting.

To ensure no confusion or misunderstanding exist of the difference between the terms "serious" and "severe," which are not synonymous, the following note of clarification is provided:

> The term "severe" is often used to describe the intensity (severity) of a specific event (as in mild, moderate, or severe myocardial infarction); the event itself, however, may be of relatively minor medical significance (such as severe headache). This is not the same as "serious," which is based on patient/event outcome or action criteria usually associated with events that pose a threat to a patient's life or functioning. Seriousness (not severity) serves as a guide for defining regulatory reporting obligations.

After reviewing the various regulatory and other definitions in use or under discussion elsewhere, the following definition is believed to encompass the spirit and meaning of them all:

> A serious adverse event (experience) or reaction is any untoward medical occurrence that at any dose:

- Results in death,
- Is life-threatening,

NOTE: The term "life-threatening" in the definition of "serious" refers to an event in which the patient was at risk of death at the time of the event; it does not refer to an event which hypothetically might have caused death if it were more severe.

> - Requires inpatient hospitalization or prolongation of existing hospitalization,

- ▪ Results in persistent or significant disability/incapacity, or
- ▪ Is a congenital anomaly/birth defect.

Medical and scientific judgment should be exercised in deciding whether expedited reporting is appropriate in other situations, such as important medical events that may not be immediately life-threatening or result in death or hospitalization but may jeopardize the patient or may require intervention to prevent one of the other outcomes listed in the definition above. These should also usually be considered serious.

Examples of such events are intensive treatment in an emergency room or at home for allergic bronchospasm; blood dyscrasias or convulsions that do not result in hospitalization; or development of drug dependency or drug abuse.

C. Expectedness of an Adverse Drug Reaction

The purpose of expedited reporting is to make regulators, investigators, and other appropriate people aware of new, important information on serious reactions. Therefore, such reporting will generally involve events previously unobserved or undocumented, and a guideline is needed on how to define an event as "unexpected" or "expected" (expected/unexpected from the perspective of previously observed, not on the basis of what might be anticipated from the pharmacological properties of a medicinal product).

As stated in the definition (II.A.3.), an "unexpected" adverse reaction is one, the nature or severity of which is not consistent with information in the relevant source document(s). Until source documents are amended, expedited reporting is required for additional occurrences of the reaction.

The following documents or circumstances will be used to determine whether an adverse event/reaction is expected:

1. For a medicinal product not yet approved for marketing in a country, a company's Investigator's Brochure will serve as the source document in that country. See section III.F. and ICH Guideline for the Investigator's Brochure.

2. Reports which add significant information on specificity or severity of a known, already documented serious ADR constitute unexpected events. For example, an event more specific or more severe than described in the Investigator's Brochure would be considered "unexpected." Specific examples would be (a) acute renal failure as a labeled ADR with a subsequent new report of interstitial nephritis and (b) hepatitis with a first report of fulminant hepatitis.

III. *STANDARDS FOR EXPEDITED REPORTING*

A. What Should be Reported?

1. Single Cases of Serious, Unexpected ADRs

All ADRs that are both serious and unexpected are subject to expedited reporting. This applies to reports from spontaneous sources and from any type of clinical or epidemiological investigation, independent of design or purpose. It also applies to cases not reported directly to a sponsor or manufacturer (for example, those found in regulatory authority generated ADR registries or in publications). The source of a report (investigation, spontaneous, other) should always be specified.

Expedited reporting of reactions that are serious but expected will ordinarily be inappropriate. Expedited reporting is also inappropriate for serious events from clinical investigations that are considered not related to study product, whether the event is expected or not. Similarly, non-serious adverse reactions, whether expected or not, will ordinarily not be subject to expedited reporting.

Information obtained by a sponsor or manufacturer on serious, unexpected reports from any source should be submitted on an expedited basis to appropriate regulatory authorities if the minimum criteria for expedited reporting can be met. See section III.B.

Causality assessment is required for clinical investigation cases. All cases judged by either the reporting health care professional or the sponsor as having a reasonable suspected causal relationship to the medicinal product qualify as ADRs. For purposes of reporting, adverse event reports associated with marketed drugs (spontaneous reports) usually imply causality.

Many terms and scales are in use to describe the degree of causality (attributability) between a medicinal product and an event, such as certainly, definitely, probably, possibly or likely related or not related. Phrases such as "plausible relationship," "suspected causality," or "causal relationship cannot be ruled out" are also invoked to describe cause and effect. However, there is currently no standard international nomenclature. The expression "reasonable causal relationship" is meant to convey in general that there are facts (evidence) or arguments to suggest a causal relationship.

2.   Other Observations

There are situations in addition to single case reports of "serious" adverse events or reactions that may necessitate rapid communication to regulatory authorities; appropriate medical and scientific judgment should be applied for each situation. In general, information that might materially influence the benefit-risk assessment of a medicinal product or that would be sufficient to consider changes in medicinal product administration or in the overall conduct of a clinical investigation represents such situations. Examples include:

a. For an "expected," serious ADR, an increase in the rate of occurrence which is judged to be clinically important.
b. A significant hazard to the patient population, such as lack of efficacy with a medicinal product used in treating life-threatening disease.
c. A major safety finding from a newly completed animal study (such as carcinogenicity).

B. Reporting Time Frames

1. Fatal or Life-Threatening Unexpected ADRs

Certain ADRs may be sufficiently alarming so as to require very rapid notification to regulators in countries where the medicinal product or indication, formulation, or population for the medicinal product are still not approved for marketing, because such reports may lead to consideration of suspension of, or other limitations to, a clinical investigation program. Fatal or life-threatening, unexpected ADRs occurring in clinical investigations qualify for very rapid reporting. Regulatory agencies should be notified (e.g., by telephone, facsimile transmission, or in writing) as soon as possible but no later than 7 calendar days after first knowledge by the sponsor that a case qualifies, followed by as complete a report as possible within 8 additional calendar days. This report should include an assessment of the importance and implication of the findings, including relevant previous experience with the same or similar medicinal products.

2. All Other Serious, Unexpected ADRs

Serious, unexpected reactions (ADRs) that are not fatal or life-threatening must be filed as soon as possible but no later than 15 calendar days after first knowledge by the sponsor that the case meets the minimum criteria for expedited reporting.

3. Minimum Criteria for Reporting

Information for final description and evaluation of a case report may not be available within the required time frames for reporting outlined above. Nevertheless, for regulatory purposes, initial reports should be submitted within the prescribed time as long as the following minimum criteria are met: an identifiable patient; a suspect medicinal product; an identifiable reporting source; and an event or outcome that can be identified as serious and unexpected, and for which, in clinical investigation cases, there is a reasonable suspected causal relationship. Follow-up information should be actively sought and submitted as it becomes available.

C. How to Report

The CIOMS-I form has been a widely accepted standard for expedited adverse event reporting. However, no matter what the form or format used, it is important that certain basic information/data elements, when available, be included with any expedited report, whether in a tabular or narrative presentation. The listing in Attachment 1 addresses those data elements regarded as desirable; if all are not available at the time of expedited reporting, efforts should be made to obtain them. See section III.B.

All reports must be sent to those regulators or other official parties requiring them (as appropriate for the local situation) in countries where the drug is under development.

D.   Managing Blinded Therapy Cases

When the sponsor and investigator are blinded to individual patient treatment (as in a double-blind study), the occurrence of a serious event requires a decision on whether to open (break) the code for the specific patient. If the investigator breaks the blind, then it is assumed the sponsor will also know the assigned treatment for that patient. Although it is advantageous to retain the blind for all patients prior to final study analysis, when a serious adverse reaction is judged reportable on an expedited basis, it is recommended that the blind be broken only for that specific patient by the sponsor even if the investigator has not broken the blind. It is also recommended that, when possible and appropriate, the blind be maintained for those persons, such as biometrics personnel, responsible for analysis and interpretation of results at the study's conclusion.

There are several disadvantages to maintaining the blind under the circumstances described which outweigh the advantages. By retaining the blind, placebo and comparator (usually a marketed product) cases are filed unnecessarily. When the blind is eventually opened, which may be many weeks or months after reporting to regulators, it must be ensured that company and regulatory data bases are revised. If the event is serious, new, and possibly related to the medicinal product, then if the Investigator's Brochure is updated, notifying relevant parties of the new information in a blinded fashion is inappropriate and possibly misleading. Moreover, breaking the blind for a single patient usually has little or no significant implications for the conduct of the clinical investigation or on the analysis of the final clinical investigation data.

However, when a fatal or other "serious" outcome is the primary efficacy endpoint in a clinical investigation, the integrity of the clinical investigation may be compromised if the blind is broken. Under these and similar circumstances, it may be appropriate to reach agreement with regulatory authorities in advance concerning serious events that would be treated as disease-related and not subject to routine expedited reporting.

E.   Miscellaneous Issues

1.   Reactions Associated with Active Comparator or Placebo Treatment

It is the sponsor's responsibility to decide whether active comparator drug reactions should be reported to the other manufacturer and/or directly to appropriate regulatory agencies. Sponsors should report such events to either the manufacturer of the active control or to appropriate regulatory agencies. Events associated with placebo will usually not satisfy the criteria for an ADR and, therefore, for expedited reporting.

2.   Products with More Than One Presentation or Use

To avoid ambiguities and uncertainties, an ADR that qualifies for expedited reporting with one presentation of a product (e.g., a dosage form, formulation, delivery system) or product use (e.g., for an indication or population), should be reported or referenced to regulatory filings across other product presentations and uses.

It is not uncommon that more than one dosage form, formulation, or delivery system (oral, IM, IV, topical, etc.) of the pharmacologically active compound(s) is under study or marketed; for these different presentations there may be some marked differences in the clinical safety profile. The same may apply for a given product used in different indications or populations (single dose vs. chronic administration, for example). Thus, "expectedness" may be product or product use specific, and separate Investigator's Brochures may be used accordingly. However, such documents are expected to cover ADR information that applies to all affected product presentations and uses. When relevant, separate discussions of pertinent product-specific or use-specific safety information will also be included.

It is recommended that any adverse drug reactions that qualify for expedited reporting observed with one product dosage form or use be cross referenced to regulatory records for all other dosage forms and uses for that product. This may result in a certain amount of overreporting or unnecessary reporting in obvious situations (for example, a report of phlebitis on IV injection sent to authorities in a country where only an oral dosage form is studied or marketed). However, underreporting is completely avoided.

3. Post-study Events

    Although such information is not routinely sought or collected by the sponsor, serious adverse events that occurred after the patient had completed a clinical study (including any protocol required post-treatment follow-up) will possibly be reported by an investigator to the sponsor. Such cases should be regarded for expedited reporting purposes as though they were study reports. Therefore, a causality assessment and determination of expectedness are needed for a decision on whether or not expedited reporting is required.

F. Informing Investigators and Ethics Committees/Institutional Review Boards of New Safety Information

International standards regarding such communication are discussed within the ICH GCP Guidelines, including the addendum on "Guideline for the Investigator's Brochure." In general, the sponsor of a study should amend the Investigator's Brochure as needed, and in accord with any local regulatory requirements, so as to keep the description of safety information updated.

IV. REFERENCE

Federal Register. Vol.60, No. 40, Wednesday, March 1, 1995, pages 1128411287.

KEY DATA ELEMENTS FOR INCLUSION IN EXPEDITED REPORTS OF SERIOUS ADVERSE DRUG REACTIONS

The following list of items has its foundation in several established precedents, including those of CIOMS-I, the WHO International Drug Monitoring Centre, and various regulatory authority forms and guidelines. Some items may not be relevant depending on the circumstances. The minimum information required for expedited reporting purposes is: an identifiable patient, the name of a suspect medicinal product, an identifiable reporting source, and an event or outcome that can be identified as serious and unexpected and for which, in clinical investigation cases, there is a reasonable suspected causal relationship. Attempts should be made to obtain follow-up information on as many other listed items pertinent to the case.

1. Patient Details:

    - Initials,
    - Other relevant identifier (clinical investigation number, for example),
    - Gender,
    - Age and/or date of birth,
    - Weight,
    - Height,

2. Suspected Medicinal Product(s):

    - Brand name as reported,
    - International Non-Proprietary Name (INN),
    - Batch number,
    - Indication(s) for which suspect medicinal product was prescribed or tested,

- Dosage form and strength,
- Daily dose and regimen (specify units - e.g., mg, mL, mg/kg),
- Route of administration,
- Starting date and time of day,
- Stopping date and time, or duration of treatment.

3. Other Treatment(s):

- For concomitant medicinal products (including non-prescription/OTC medicinal products) and non-medicinal product therapies, provide the same information as for the suspected product.

4. Details of Suspected Adverse Drug Reaction(s):

- Full description of reaction(s) including body site and severity, as well as the criterion (or criteria) for regarding the report as serious should be given. In addition to a description of the reported signs and symptoms, whenever possible, attempts should be made to establish a specific diagnosis for the reaction.
- Start date (and time) of onset of reaction,
- Stop date (and time) or duration of reaction,
- Dechallenge and rechallenge information,
- Setting (e.g., hospital, out-patient clinic, home, nursing home),
- Outcome: Information on recovery and any sequelae; what specific tests and/or treatment may have been required and their results; for a fatal outcome, cause of death and a comment on its possible relationship to the suspected reaction should be provided. Any autopsy or other post-mortem findings (including a coroner's report) should also be provided when available. Other information: anything relevant to facilitate assessment of the case, such as medical history including allergy, drug or alcohol abuse; family history; findings from special investigations.

5. Details on Reporter of Event (Suspected ADR):

- Name,
- Address,
- Telephone number,
- Profession (specialty).

6. Administrative and Sponsor/Company Details:

- Source of report: Was it spontaneous, from a clinical investigation (provide details), from the literature (provide copy), other?
- Date event report was first received by sponsor/manufacturer,
- Country in which event occurred,
- Type of report filed to authorities: initial or follow-up (first, second, etc.),
- Name and address of sponsor/manufacturer/company,
- Name, address, telephone number, and FAX number of contact person in reporting company or institution,
- Identifying regulatory code or number for marketing authorization dossier or clinical investigation process for the suspected product (for example IND or CTX number, NDA number),
- Sponsor/manufacturer's identification number for the case (This number should be the same for the initial and follow-up reports on the same case).

Printed in the United States
by Baker & Taylor Publisher Services